# ICD-10-CM
# Coder Training Manual
# 2013

**Prepared by the
HIM Solutions Team
American Health Information
Management Association**

**Contributing Authors
Kathryn DeVault, RHIA, CCS, CCS-P
Ann Barta, MSA, RHIA
Melanie Endicott, MBA/HCM, RHIA, CDIP, CCS, CCS-P**

AHIMA
PRESS

AHIMA Product No.: AC206813

ISBN: 978-1-58426-389-0

The websites listed in this book were current and valid as of the date of publication. However, webpage addresses and the information on them may change or disappear at any time and for any number of reasons. The user is encouraged to perform his or her own general web searches to locate any URLs listed here that are no longer valid.

AHIMA Staff:
Angie Comfort, RHIT, CDIP, CCS, Technical Review
Katie Greenock, MS, Editorial and Production Coordinator
Jessica Block, MA, Assistant Editor
Jason O. Malley, Director, Creative Content Development
Pamela Woolf, Managing Editor

American Health Information Management Association
233 North Michigan Avenue, 21st Floor
Chicago, Illinois 60601-5809
www.ahima.org

# Contents

# About the Authors

**Kathryn DeVault, RHIA, CCS, CCS-P,** is a director of HIM Solutions for AHIMA. In her role, she provides professional expertise to AHIMA members, the media, and outside organizations on professional practice issues. In addition, she authors materials for and supports AHIMA online coding education, including the AHIMA Coding Basics program. Ms. DeVault also serves as a technical advisor for the association on ICD-9-CM, ICD-10, and CPT coding publications. Ms. DeVault also serves as author and faculty for the AHIMA ICD-10-CM/PCS Academies.

Prior to joining AHIMA in 2008, Ms. DeVault served as data quality analyst for coding in a regional healthcare system. For the past eight years, she has been a coding educator at a local community college. Ms. DeVault has authored many articles and has presented numerous seminars and educational sessions on coding and HIM-related topics.

As an AHIMA member, Ms. DeVault has participated in numerous leadership roles at both the state and regional level through the Colorado Health Information Management Association. She received her bachelor's degree in liberal arts from the University of Colorado.

**Ann Barta, MSA, RHIA** is a director of HIM Solutions for AHIMA. In her role, she provides professional expertise to AHIMA members, the media, and outside organizations on professional practice issues. In addition, she authors materials for and supports AHIMA online coding education, including the AHIMA Coding Basics program. Ms. Barta also serves as faculty for the AHIMA ICD-10-CM/PCS Academies.

Prior to joining AHIMA, Ms. Barta participated in a one-year contract between the AHIMA Foundation of Research and Education and Centers for Medicare and Medicaid Services (CMS) to determine potential impacts to CMS when converting from ICD-9-CM to ICD-10-CM/PCS coding systems. Prior to that, Ms. Barta served as a corporate coding manager for a large healthcare system. She has more than 30 years experience as an HIM director and coding consultant. She has been an educator of coding and HIM for more than 15 years, served as an associate dean for health sciences, and was system coordinator for an RHIT program.

As an AHIMA member, Ms. Barta participated in various leadership positions. She has served on various RHIT Program Advisory Boards. Additionally, she was actively involved with the Illinois Health Information Management Association, serving on the Education Committee and as a state coding instructor with the implementation of ICD-9-CM. Ms. Barta received her master of science in health services administration from Central Michigan University in Mt. Pleasant.

**Melanie Endicott, MBA/HCM, RHIA, CDIP, CCS, CCS-P,** is a director of HIM Solutions for AHIMA providing professional expertise to AHIMA members on professional practice issue. She also authors and supports AHIMA online coding education, including the Coding Basics program. Ms. Endicott is also an AHIMA ICD-10-CM/PCS Academy faculty member.

Prior to joining AHIMA in 2004, Ms. Endicott served as health information analyst for coding in a large acute-care facility. She has been an educator of health information technology and health information administration for several years at several colleges and universities. She has presented numerous seminars and educational sessions on coding and HIM-related topics at the local, state, and regional levels.

As an AHIMA member, Ms. Endicott also participated in numerous leadership roles at both the state and regional level through the Washington State Health Information Management Association. She received her bachelor's degree in health information management from Carroll College and her master's degree in business administration and healthcare management from the University of Phoenix.

# Acknowledgments

The exercises in this book were created using several AHIMA resources as a base. All of the adapted materials underwent a vigorous review to bring them into alignment with the latest versions of the ICD-10-CM code sets and guidelines which were available at the time of publication.

The author team adapted many of the application exercises in this book from case scenarios originally created by Anita Hazelwood, MLS, RHIA, FAHIMA and Carol Venable, MPH, RHIA, FAHIMA. The authors also would like to thank Sue Bowman, RHIA, CCS, FAHIMA for her contribution to the content and review of this publication. In addition, the authors would like to thank June Bronnert, RHIA, CCS, CCS-P; Ann Zeisset, RHIT, CCS, CCS-P; Anita Majerowicz, MS, RHIA; and Lynn Kuehn, MS, RHIA, CCS-P, FAHIMA for their contributions.

# Preface to the Training Manual

On January 16, 2009, the US Department of Health and Human Services (HHS) published a Final Rule for the adoption of ICD-10-CM and ICD-10-PCS code sets to replace the 30-year-old ICD-9-CM code sets under rules 45 CFR Parts 160 and 162 of the Health Insurance Portability and Accountability Act of 1996 (HIPAA). The initial compliance date for the two classification sets was established as October 1, 2013 and this has subsequently been revised with an updated compliance date of October 1, 2014. A second rule related to the HIPAA transaction standards—X12 version 5010 and NCPDP version D.0—establishes earlier effective dates. The HIPAA transactions software must be updated to accommodate the use of the ICD-10-CM and ICD-10-PCS code sets by January 1, 2012 with the exception of Medicaid Pharmacy Subrogation Transactions, which have an effective date of January 1, 2013.

To read the final rules published in the *Federal Register*, please go to the following websites:

- Modifications to the Health Insurance Portability and Accountability Act (HIPAA) Electronic Transaction Standards:
  http://edocket.access.gpo.gov/2009/pdf/E9-740.pdf
- HIPAA Administrative Simplification: Modifications to Medical Data Code Set Standards To Adopt ICD–10–CM and ICD–10–PCS:
  http://edocket.access.gpo.gov/2009/pdf/E9-743.pdf
- ICD–10–CM/PCS final compliance date:
  http://www.gpo.gov/fdsys/pkg/FR-2012-09-05/pdf/2012-21238.pdf

The adoption of ICD-10-CM (diagnoses) will affect all components of the healthcare industry. However, the adoption of ICD-10-PCS will affect only those components of the healthcare industry that currently utilize ICD-9-CM Volume 3—inpatient procedures. Therefore, CPT® and HCPCS Level II will continue to be used for reporting physician and other professional services in addition to procedures performed in hospital outpatient departments and other outpatient facilities.

The three key issues HHS believes necessitate the need to update from ICD-9-CM to ICD-10-CM and ICD-10-PCS are

- ICD-9-CM is out of date and running out of space for new codes.
- ICD-10 is the international standard to report and monitor diseases and mortality, making it important for the United States to adopt ICD-10-based classifications for reporting and surveillance.
- ICD codes are core elements of many health information technology (HIT) systems, making the conversion to ICD-10-CM/PCS necessary to fully realize benefits of HIT adoption.

The use of ICD-10-CM will offer greater detail and granularity and will greatly enhance HHS's capability to measure quality outcomes, such as the quality performance outcome measures used in the hospital pay-for-reporting program. The greater detail and granularity of ICD-10-CM/PCS will also provide more precision for claims-based, value-based purchase initiatives such as the hospital-acquired condition (HAC) payment policy.

In addition, the transition to ICD-10-CM/PCS will ultimately facilitate realizing the benefits of using interoperability standards specified by the Healthcare Information Technology Standards Panel (HITSP), including SNOMED CT®. The benefits of using SNOMED CT increase if such use is linked to classification systems such as ICD-10-CM and ICD-10-PCS. Mapping would be used to link SNOMED CT to these new code sets, and plans are underway to develop these maps.

# How to Use This Manual

The AHIMA Academy for ICD-10-CM Trainers is primarily designed to prepare individuals to train others in ICD-10-CM through course content that focuses on instruction in the code set. The *ICD-10-CM Coder Training Manual 2013* is designed to be used by students who are trained by AHIMA Academy ICD-10-CM trainers to build upon their basic knowledge of ICD-10-CM fundamentals. Although the implementation date for ICD-10-CM/PCS is several years away, it is necessary that individuals responsible for training are fully knowledgeable of the code sets in order to prepare students and the workforce for the transition. Transitioning curriculum from ICD-9-CM to ICD-10-CM/PCS will present unique challenges for academicians. Educating the workforce will also require that the healthcare industry begin planning and preparing for the new code sets.

The content of the *ICD-10-CM Coder Training Manual 2013* is based on the August, 2012 release of the *International Classification of Diseases, Tenth Revision, Clinical Modification* (ICD-10-CM), which can be downloaded from the following website: http://www.cdc.gov/nchs/icd/icd10cm.htm.

The ICD-10-CM Coder *Training Manual 2013* contains many references to and explanations of ICD-10-CM coding guidelines and conventions. It includes ICD-10-CM coding exercises at the basic, intermediate, and advanced level as well as beginner, intermediate, and advanced coding exercises. These coding exercises emphasize all aspects of the coding classification system so students can apply their knowledge of coding principles and definitions. Answers to the coding exercises are provided.

Students should recognize that additional, self-directed study will be required to master the guidelines and principles of ICD-10-CM coding beyond the materials provided in this manual. In addition, many students will require additional coursework to increase their level of knowledge in anatomy, physiology, pathophysiology, pharmacology, and medical terminology. Because ICD-10-CMS requires a stronger background in the biomedical sciences, instructors should develop plans for assessing their students' strengths/weaknesses in these areas. Identifying students' learning needs and levels of knowledge is crucial to preparing a solid educational transition plan.

In addition to this text, students of the AHIMA Academy will use the 2013 *ICD-10-CM: The Complete Official Draft Code Set* code book (Optum) to complete the practice exercises.

# Introduction: ICD-10-CM Overview

# Section 1 – Introduction to the ICD-10-CM Classification System

## *History*

The *International Classification of Diseases, Tenth Revision, Clinical Modification (ICD-10-CM)* is the United States' clinical modification to the World Health Organization's (WHO) *International Classification of Diseases, Tenth Revision (ICD-10)*. ICD-10 was adopted by the World Health Assembly in 1990. Following the publication of ICD-10, a number of countries performed an analysis to determine if the WHO classification would meet their needs given the changes to the roles of ICD since the *Ninth Revision*.

The first modification to ICD-10 was published in 1998. The Australian National Centre for Classification in Health (NCCH) published the *International Statistical Classification of Diseases and Related Health Problems, Tenth Revision, Australian Modification* (ICD-10-AM). Subsequent editions have been made available every two years.

In 2001, the Canadian Institute for Health Information (CIHI), through the work of an Expert Panel, published the *International Statistical Classification of Diseases and Related Health Problems, Tenth Revision, Canada* (ICD-10-CA).

The United States remains the only industrialized nation that has not yet implemented ICD-10 (or a clinical modification) for morbidity, meaning diseases or causes of illness typically coded in a healthcare facility. Since 1999, however, the United States has used ICD-10 for mortality reporting—the coding of death certificates (typically done by a vital statistics office, not the healthcare facility). Implementing ICD-10-CM will maintain data comparability internationally and between mortality and morbidity data in the United States.

> **Activity – History of ICD-10**
> To learn more about the processes involved with ICD-10, visit the World Health Organization website (http://www.who.int/classifications/icd/en/).
>
> Review the information on ICD-10 with special attention to the implementation of ICD-10 (http://www.who/int/classifications/icd/implementation/en/index.html).

> **NOTE:** There is an ICD-10 training tool on the WHO website that you are welcome to peruse; however, remember that this information pertains to ICD-10 and not to the US modification of ICD-10-CM.

## *Development of ICD-10-CM*

In 1994, under the leadership of the National Center for Health Statistics (NCHS), the United States began their process of determining whether an ICD-10 modification should be developed. NCHS awarded a contract to the Center for Health Policy Studies to decide if a clinical modification was necessary. A Technical Advisory Panel (TAP) was formed and their recommendation was to create a clinical modification. In 1997, the entire draft of the Tabular List of ICD-10-CM and the preliminary crosswalk between ICD-9-CM and ICD-10-CM were made available on the NCHS website for public comments. The public comment period ran from December 1997 through February 1998. Since that time revisions were based on further study and the comments submitted. Draft versions of ICD-10-CM were made available in 2002, 2007, 2009, 2010, 2011, 2012, and 2013. One last limited code update will be made to the

ICD-10-CM code set in 2014. Beginning October 1, 2015, ICD-10-CM will have regular annual updates which go into effect on October 1 of each year.

While ICD-10 provides many more categories for diseases and other health-related conditions than previous revisions, the clinical modifications thus far to ICD-10 offer a higher level of specificity by including separate codes for laterality and additional characters for expanded detail. In addition, other changes include combining etiology and manifestations, poisoning and external cause, or diagnosis and symptoms into a single code. ICD-10-CM also provides code titles and language that complement accepted clinical practice. ICD-10-CM codes have the potential to reveal more about quality of care, so that data can be used in a more meaningful way to better understand complications, better design clinically robust algorithms, and better track the outcomes of care. ICD-10-CM incorporates greater specificity and clinical detail to provide information for clinical decision making and outcome research.

The long-awaited official Notice of Proposed Rule Making (NPRM) related to the adoption of the ICD-10-CM and ICD-10-PCS classifications was published in the Federal Register on August 22, 2008. Additional information is available on the CMS website. On January 16, 2009, the Centers for Medicare and Medicaid Services (CMS) published a Health and Human Services (HHS) compliance date of October 1, 2013, for the two code sets. This compliance date has subsequently been delayed until October 1, 2014, and is based on the date of discharge for inpatient claims and the date of service for outpatient claims.

> **Note:** Additional information about the development of ICD-10-CM and the final rule can be found on the CMS website (https://www.cms.gov/icd10/).

This rule will modify two of the medical data code set standards adopted in the Transactions and Code Sets final rule published in the *Federal Register*. It would also implement certain provisions of the Administrative Simplification subtitle of the Health Insurance Portability and Accountability Act (HIPAA) of 1996. Specifically, the rule would modify the standard code sets for coding diagnoses and inpatient hospital procedures by concurrently adopting the *International Classification of Diseases, Tenth Revision, Clinical Modification* (ICD-10-CM) for diagnosis coding, and the *International Classification of Diseases, Tenth Revision, Procedure Coding System* (ICD-10-PCS) for inpatient hospital procedure coding. These new codes will replace the *International Classification of Diseases, Ninth Revision, Clinical Modification* (ICD-9-CM) Volumes 1 and 2 and the *International Classification of Diseases, Ninth Revision, Clinical Modification* (CM) Volume 3 for diagnosis and procedure codes respectively.

> **Note:** CPT® will continue to be used by all providers currently using it.

## *Organizational and Structural Changes in ICD-10-CM*

ICD-10-CM represents a significant improvement over ICD-9-CM. ICD-10-CM continues to have the same hierarchical structure as ICD-9-CM where the first three characters are the category of the code and all codes within the same category have similar traits. Although the hierarchical structure is the same, differences are seen in the organization of ICD-10-CM, including
- ICD-10-CM consists of 21 chapters compared to 17 chapters in ICD-9-CM
- ICD-9-CM's V and E code supplemental classifications are incorporated into the main classification in ICD-10-CM
- Diseases and conditions of the sense organs (eyes and ears) have been separated from the nervous system diseases and conditions and have their own chapters in ICD-10-CM

- To reflect current medical knowledge, certain diseases have been reclassified (or reassigned) to a more appropriate chapter in ICD-10-CM. For example, gout has been reclassified from the endocrine chapter in ICD-9-CM to the musculoskeletal chapter in ICD-10-CM
- In contrast to ICD-9-CM, which classifies injuries by type, ICD-10-CM groups injuries first by specific site (e.g., head, arm, leg), and then by type of injury (e.g., fracture, open wound)
- Postoperative complications have been moved to procedure-specific body system chapters
- ICD-10-CM codes are alphanumeric and can be up to seven characters in length; ICD-9-CM codes are only three to five characters in length
- ICD-10-CM includes full code titles for all codes (no reference back to common fourth and fifth digits)
- Addition of a sixth character in some chapters
- Addition of seventh characters for obstetrics, injuries, and external causes of injuries
- Addition of placeholder X

## New Features in ICD-10-CM

The numerous new features in ICD-10-CM allow for a greater level of specificity and clinical detail. These new features include

- Combination codes for conditions and common symptoms or manifestations

---

*Examples:*
- ➤ E10.21, Type 1 diabetes mellitus with diabetic nephropathy
- ➤ I25.110, Atherosclerotic heart disease of native coronary artery with unstable angina pectoris
- ➤ K50.112, Crohn's disease of large intestine with intestinal obstruction

---

- Combination codes for poisonings and external causes

---

*Examples:*
- ➤ T36.0X1D, Poisoning by penicillins, accidental (unintentional), subsequent encounter
- ➤ T42.4X5A, Adverse effect of benzodiazepines, initial encounter

---

- Added laterality

---

*Examples:*
- ➤ H60.332, Swimmer's ear, left ear
- ➤ M94.211, Chondromalacia, right shoulder
- ➤ S40.259A, Superficial foreign body of unspecified shoulder, initial encounter

---

- Added seventh-characters for episode of care

---

*Examples:*
- ➢ M80.051A, Age-related osteoporosis with current pathological fracture, right femur, initial encounter for fracture
- ➢ S06.0X1A, Concussion with loss of consciousness of 30 minutes or less, initial encounter
- ➢ S52.132B, Displaced fracture of neck of left radius, initial encounter for open fracture Type I or II or initial encounter for open fracture NOS

---

- Expanded codes (injuries, diabetes, alcohol and substance abuse, postoperative complications)

---

*Examples:*
- ➢ E11.341, Type 2 diabetes mellitus with severe nonproliferative diabetic retinopathy with macular edema
- ➢ F14.221, Cocaine dependence with intoxication delirium
- ➢ K91.71, Accidental puncture and laceration of a digestive system organ or structure during a digestive system procedure

---

- Inclusion of trimesters in obstetrics codes (and elimination of fifth digits for episode of care)

---

*Examples:*
- ➢ O10.012, Pre-existing essential hypertension complicating pregnancy, second trimester
- ➢ O99.013, Anemia complicating pregnancy, third trimester

---

- Changes in time frames specified in certain codes

---

*Examples:*
- ➢ Acute myocardial infarction—time period changed from 8 weeks to 4 weeks
- ➢ Time frame for abortion versus fetal death changed from 22 weeks to 20 weeks

---

- Added standard definitions for two types of "excludes" notes

---

*Examples:*
- ➢ *Excludes1* note indicates "not coded here." The code being excluded is never used with the code. The two conditions cannot occur together.
  *Example:* B06, Rubella (German measles) has an *Excludes1* of congenital rubella (P35.0)
- ➢ *Excludes2* note indicates "not included here." The excluded condition is not part of the condition represented by the code. It is acceptable to use both codes together if the patient has both conditions.
  *Example:* J04.0, Acute laryngitis has an *Excludes2* of chronic laryngitis (J37.0)

---

**Activity – New Features in ICD-10-CM**
Answer each of the following questions.

1. True or false? V and E codes are supplemental classifications in ICD-10-CM.  F

2. True or false? In ICD-10-CM, injuries are grouped by anatomical site rather than  T injury category.

3. How are obstetric cases classified in ICD-10-CM?  Trimesters

4. What is the maximum number of characters in ICD-10-CM?  7

5. How many chapters does ICD-10-CM contain?  21

---

## *General Equivalence Mappings (GEMs)*

Mappings between ICD-9-CM and ICD-10-CM classification systems have been developed to facilitate the transition from one code set to another. Public domain diagnosis code reference mapping files referred to as Diagnosis Code Set General Equivalence Mappings (GEMs) have been released by NCHS. There are two GEMs files available allowing for bidirectional mappings, ICD-9-CM to ICD-10-CM and ICD-10-CM to ICD-9-CM. The GEMs, along with documentation and a user's guide, are available on the NCHS website (http://www.cdc.gov/nchs/icd/icd10cm.htm) and the CMS website (http://www.cms.hhs.gov/ICD10).

---

**Appropriate Usage of GEMs:**
- Convert multiple databases from ICD-9-CM to ICD-10-CM
- Variety of research applications involving trend data

**Inappropriate Usage of GEMs:**
- Crosswalks
  *There is not a one-to-one match between ICD-9-CM and ICD-10-CM codes, for a multitude of reasons (e.g., new concepts in ICD-10-CM, a single ICD-9-CM code may map to multiple ICD-10-CM codes).*

---

**Optional Resources:**

Effectiveness of ICD-10-CM in Capturing Public Health Diseases:
http://library.ahima.org/xpedio/groups/public/documents/ahima/bok1_034294.pdf

ICD-10-CM Enhancements:
http://library.ahima.org/xpedio/groups/public/documents/ahima/bok1_042626.hcsp

ICD-10-CM Primer:
http://library.ahima.org/xpedio/groups/public/documents/ahima/bok1_038084.hcsp

Mortality Coding Marks 10 Years of ICD-10:
http://library.ahima.org/xpedio/groups/public/documents/ahima/bok1_043992.hcsp

Putting the ICD-10-CM/PCS GEMs into Practice:
http://library.ahima.org/xpedio/groups/public/documents/ahima/bok1_046756.hcsp

Why ICD-10 is Worth the Trouble:
http://library.ahima.org/xpedio/groups/public/documents/ahima/bok1_036866.hcsp

## *Code Structure*

The first character of an ICD-10-CM code is an alphabetic letter. All the letters of the alphabet are utilized with the exception of the letter U, which has been reserved by the WHO for the provisional assignment of new diseases of uncertain etiology (U00-U49) and for bacterial agents resistant to antibiotics (U80-U89). Some conditions in ICD-10-CM are not limited to the use of a single letter. For instance, neoplasm codes may begin with the letter C or D. Table 1.1 compares characteristics of ICD-10-CM and ICD-9-CM.

**Table 1.1. Comparing ICD-9-CM and ICD-10-CM**

| ICD-10-CM differs from ICD-9-CM in its organization and structure, code composition, and level of detail. ||
|---|---|
| **ICD-9-CM** | **ICD-10-CM** |
| <ul><li>Consists of three to five digits</li><li>First digit is numeric or alpha (E or V)</li><li>Second, third, fourth, and fifth digits are numeric</li><li>Always at least three digits</li><li>Decimal placed after the first three digits</li><li>Alpha characters are not case-sensitive</li></ul> | <ul><li>Consists of three to seven characters</li><li>First character is alpha</li><li>All letters used except U</li><li>Character 2 always numeric</li><li>Characters 3 through 7 can be alpha or numeric</li><li>Decimal placed after the first three characters</li><li>Alpha characters are not case-sensitive</li></ul> |

**Code Structure of ICD-10-CM versus ICD-9-CM**

ICD-10-CM codes may consist of up to seven characters, with the seventh character representing visit encounter or sequelae for injuries and external causes.

| ICD-9-CM Code Format | ICD-10-CM Code Format |
|---|---|
| X X X . X X <br><br> category — etiology, anatomic site, manifestation | X X X . X X X X <br><br> category — etiology, anatomic site, severity — extension |

**Activity – ICD-10-CM Code Structure Changes**
To become more familiar with the differences between ICD-9-CM and ICD-10-CM, go to the ICD-10-CM Tabular List, review the following entries, compare the ICD-10-CM codes to the ICD-9-CM codes, and identify their differences.

| ICD-10-CM | ICD-9-CM |
|-----------|----------|
| L03.313   | 682.2    |
| S42.311K  | 733.82   |
| T45.2X5A  | E933.5   |

# Organization and Structure of ICD-10-CM

## Alphabetic Index

The Alphabetic Index is divided into two parts—the Index to Diseases and Injuries and the Index to External Causes. Similar to ICD-9-CM, within the Index of Diseases and Injury there is a Neoplasm Table and a Table of Drugs and Chemicals.

The Alphabetic Index in ICD-10-CM is formatted the same way as the Index in ICD-9-CM. Main terms set in boldface are listed in alphabetical order. Then, indented beneath the main term, any applicable subterm or essential modifier will be shown in their own alphabetic list. The indented subterm is always read in combination with the main term. Nonessential modifiers appear in parentheses and do not affect the code number assigned. The "-" at the end of an Index entry indicates that additional characters are required.

> *Example:*
> **Aberrant (congenital)** – *see also* Malposition, congenital
> - adrenal gland Q89.1
> - artery (peripheral) Q27.8
> - - basilar NEC Q28.1
> - - cerebral Q28.3
> - breast Q83.8

*[handwritten: from the Tabular]*

> **Coding Tip:** These codes would be read:
> Q89.1, Congenital malformations of adrenal gland
> Q27.8, Other specified congenital malformations of peripheral vascular system
> Q28.1, Other malformations of precerebral vessels
> Q28.3, Other malformation of cerebral vessels
> Q83.8, Other congenital malformations of breast

Morphology Codes – Morphology codes are no longer listed in the Alphabetic Index alongside the descriptors and standard ICD-10-CM codes. Additionally, the Morphology codes no longer have a separate appendix in ICD-10-CM as in ICD-9-CM.

*[handwritten: Neoplasms]*

> **Note:** The following note appears in the Tabular List at the beginning of Chapter 2: Neoplasms.
> **Morphology [Histology]**
> Chapter 2 classifies neoplasms primarily by site (topography), with broad groupings for behavior, malignant, in situ, benign, etc. The Table of Neoplasms should be used to identify the correct topography code. In a few cases, such as for malignant melanoma and certain neuroendocrine tumors, the morphology (histologic type) is included in the category and codes.

*[handwritten: Topography → site]*

Manifestation Codes – ICD-10-CM Alphabetic Index includes the suggestion of some manifestation codes in the same manner as ICD-9-CM, by including the code as a second code, show in brackets, directly after the underlying or etiology code (which should always be reported first).

---

*Example:*
**Chorioretinitis** – *see also* Inflammation, chorioretinal, disseminated
  - Egyptian B76.9 [D63.8]
  - histoplasmic B39.9 [H32]

---

**Activity – Alphabetic Index**
To become more familiar with the ICD-10-CM Alphabetic Index to Diseases, review the following entries in the ICD-10-CM code book. If you do not have a code book, download the Index file from NCHS's website (http://www.cdc.gov/nchs/icd/icd10cm.htm). Compare the ICD-10-CM Alphabetic Index entries to the ICD-9-CM Alphabetic Index entries for the same terms and identify their similarities.

| Main term: | Adenofibroma | | |
|---|---|---|---|
| Main term: | Aftercare | Subterm: | involving |
| Main term: | Anemia | Subterm: | deficiency |
| | | Subterm: | Diamond-Blackfan |
| Main term: | Failure, failed | Subterm: | heart |
| Main term: | Pregnancy | Subterm: | complicated by |
| Main term: | Stone(s) | | |

## Tabular List

The ICD-10-CM Tabular List is divided into 21 chapters. For some chapters, the body or organ system is the axis of the classification. Other chapters, such as Chapter 1: Certain infectious and parasitic diseases, group together conditions by etiology or nature of the disease process. ICD-9-CM has a single chapter for Diseases of the Nervous System and Sense Organs whereas ICD-10-CM places these conditions into three separate chapters. ICD-10-CM also does not separate out the ICD-9-CM codes that explain the External Causes of Injury and Poisonings (E codes) and the Factors Influencing Health Status and Contact with Health Services (V codes) from the core classification.

The order of the ICD-10-CM chapters is a bit different from ICD-9-CM. In ICD-10-CM, disorders of the immune mechanism are included with Diseases of the blood and blood-forming organs. In contrast, the immunity disorders are found in the ICD-9-CM chapter for Endocrine, Nutritional and Metabolic Diseases. In addition, certain chapters are reordered. The ICD-10-CM codes for Diseases of the skin and subcutaneous tissue (Chapter 12) and Diseases of the musculoskeletal system and connective tissue (Chapter 13) follow the chapter for Diseases of the digestive system. Next are chapters for Diseases of the genitourinary system (Chapter 14), Pregnancy, childbirth and the puerperium (Chapter 15), Certain conditions originating in the perinatal period (Chapter 16), and Congenital malformations, deformations and chromosomal abnormalities (Chapter 17).

---

**Note:** Within a number of ICD-10-CM chapters, category restructuring and code reorganization have occurred resulting in the classification of certain diseases and disorders different than what is currently seen in ICD-9-CM.

---

The 21 chapters of the ICD-10-CM classification system are
1. Certain infectious and parasitic diseases (A00-B99)
2. Neoplasms (C00-D49)
3. Diseases of the blood and blood-forming organs and certain disorders involving the immune mechanism (D50-D89)
4. Endocrine, nutritional and metabolic disorders (E00-E89)
5. Mental, behavioral and neurodevelopmental disorders (F01-F99)
6. Diseases of the nervous system (G00-G99)
7. Diseases of the eye and adnexa (H00-H59)
8. Diseases of the ear and mastoid process (H60-H95)
9. Diseases of the circulatory system (I00-I99)
10. Diseases of the respiratory system (J00-J99)
11. Diseases of the digestive system (K00-K95)
12. Diseases of the skin and subcutaneous tissue (L00-L99)
13. Diseases of the musculoskeletal system and connective tissue (M00-M99)
14. Diseases of the genitourinary system (N00-N99)
15. Pregnancy, childbirth and the puerperium (O00-O9A)
16. Certain conditions originating in the perinatal period (P00-P96)
17. Congenital malformations, deformations and chromosomal abnormalities (Q00-Q99)
18. Symptoms, signs and abnormal clinical and laboratory findings, not elsewhere classified (R00-R99)
19. Injury, poisoning and certain other consequences of external causes (S00-T88)
20. External causes of morbidity (V00-Y99)
21. Factors influencing health status and contact with health services (Z00-Z99)

Chapters are further subdivided into subchapters (blocks) that contain three character categories and, similar to ICD-9-CM categories, form the foundation of the code. Each chapter in the Tabular List of ICD-10-CM begins with a summary of the blocks to provide an overview of the categories within the chapter. For example

---

Chapter 7: Diseases of the eye and adnexa (H00-H59)
This chapter contains the following blocks:

| | |
|---|---|
| H00-H05 | Disorders of eyelid, lacrimal system and orbit |
| H10-H11 | Disorders of conjunctiva |
| H15-H22 | Disorders of sclera, cornea, iris and ciliary body |
| H25-H28 | Disorders of lens |
| H30-H36 | Disorders of choroid and retina |
| H40-H42 | Glaucoma |
| H43-H44 | Disorders of vitreous body and globe |
| H46-H47 | Disorders of optic nerve and visual pathways |
| H49-H52 | Disorders of ocular muscles, binocular movement, accommodation and refraction |
| H53-H54 | Visual disturbances and blindness |
| H55-H57 | Other disorders of eye and adnexa |
| H59 | Intraoperative and postprocedural complications and disorders of eye and adnexa, not elsewhere classified |

---

Most, but not all, categories are further subdivided into four- or five-character subcategories. If a category is not further subdivided it is considered to be a valid code, such as P90, Convulsions of newborn.

The fourth character 8, when placed after a decimal point (.8), is used to indicate some "other" specified category, and the fourth character 9 placed after a decimal point (.9) is usually reserved for an unspecified condition. This represents another classification modification with the separation of Not Elsewhere Classified (NEC) and Not Otherwise Specified (NOS) codes. ICD-9-CM sometimes combines these two into a single code. In ICD-10-CM, the Other Specified and Unspecified each have their own code.

---

*Examples:*
  ➢ K52.89, Other specified noninfective gastroenteritis and colitis
  ➢ K52.9, Non-infective gastroenteritis and colitis, unspecified

---

Five- and six-character codes provide even greater specificity or additional information about the condition being coded. Similar to ICD-9-CM, ICD-10-CM codes must be used to the highest number of characters available or to the highest level of specificity. When a category has been subdivided into four-, five-, or six-character codes, the code assigned must represent the highest level of specificity represented within ICD-10-CM.

Certain categories have an additional seventh character. The seventh character must always be the seventh and final character of the code. When the code contains fewer than seven characters, placeholder X must be used to fill in the empty character(s).

---

*Example:* The code for "Exposure to supersonic waves" is a four-character code (W42.0) that requires a seventh character to describe whether this is the initial or subsequent encounter, or sequela. If this were the initial encounter, this code is written as W42.0XXA.

---

**Tabular List – Activity 1**

To become more familiar with the draft ICD-10-CM Tabular List of Diseases and Injuries, review the following entries in the ICD-10-CM code book. If you do not have a code book, download the Tabular file from the NCHS website (http://www.cdc.gov/nchs/icd/icd10cm.htm).

- Find code A54.22, Gonococcal prostatitis. Compare it to code 098.12 in ICD-9-CM.
- Locate codes C41.9, Malignant neoplasm of bone and articular cartilage, unspecified and M90.60, Osteitis deformans in neoplastic disease, unspecified site. Compare codes to 170.9 and 731.1 in ICD-9-CM.

**Tabular List – Activity 2**

To gain a better understanding of the general classification modifications made to ICD-10-CM, open the ICD-10-CM Tabular List, locate the ICD-10-CM categories, and find the associated ICD-9-CM category. Identify the similarities and the differences.

| ICD-10-CM | ICD-9-CM |
| --- | --- |
| E10-E13 | 250 |
| M10 | 274 |
| D80 | 279 |

Another structural similarity is the placement of notes in the ICD-10-CM Tabular List. As in ICD-9-CM, they are located at the beginning of chapters or any of the subdivisions that follow. Their position is important in that the notes that appear at the beginning of a chapter apply to all the categories contained within it. The same rule applies to notes found at the other subdivision levels.

**Tabular List – Activity 3**

To view examples of notes, go to the Tabular List:

- Locate the note at the beginning of Chapter 18: Symptoms, signs and abnormal clinical and laboratory findings (R00-R99) and compare the note to the note found at the beginning of Chapter 16: Symptoms, Signs and Ill-Defined Conditions (780-799) in ICD-9-CM.
- Find the note for the subchapter on Neoplasms of Uncertain Behavior (D37-D48) and review it against the one found for Neoplasms of Uncertain Behavior (235-238) in ICD-9-CM.

## *Classification Changes to Chapters 5, 19, and 20*

ICD-10 reorganized Chapters 5, 19, and 20, which are integrated into ICD-10-CM.

Chapter 5: Mental and behavioral disorders – This chapter contains more subchapters, categories, and subcategories and codes than ICD-9-CM. Consequently when comparing ICD-10-CM to ICD-9-CM some disorders are classified differently and greater clinical detail is obtainable.

---

*Example:*
ICD-9-CM        Chapter 5: Mental Disorders (290-319)
ICD-10-CM      Chapter 5: Mental, behavioral and neurodevelopmental disorders (F01-F99)

---

*Examples:*
  ➢ F10.251, Alcohol dependence with alcohol-induced psychotic disorder with hallucinations
  ➢ F17.213, Nicotine dependence, cigarettes, with withdrawal

---

Chapter 19: Injury, poisoning and certain other consequences of external causes – A significant modification was made to the classification of injuries with the publication of ICD-10 and therefore ICD-10-CM. Specific types of injuries found in categories S00-S99 of Chapter 19 of ICD-10-CM are arranged by body region beginning with the head and concluding with the ankle and foot. However, effects of a foreign body, burns, and frostbite are not classified in the body region groups. This chapter also includes codes for poisoning, adverse effects, and other consequences of external causes. In contrast, the type of injury is the axis of classification for the ICD-9-CM Chapter 17: Injury and Poisoning.

---

*Example:*
ICD-9-CM        Chapter 17: Injury and Poisoning (800-999)
ICD-10-CM      Chapter 19: Injury, poisoning and certain other consequences of external causes
                        (S00-T88)

---

*Examples:*
  ➢ S32.111A, Minimally displaced Zone I fracture of sacrum, initial encounter for
                        closed fracture
  ➢ T22.151D, Burn of first degree of right shoulder, subsequent encounter
  ➢ T45.516A, Underdosing of anticoagulant, initial encounter

---

Chapter 20: External causes of morbidity – Codes for external causes are no longer located in a supplemental classification in ICD-10-CM. The causes currently located in the ICD-9-CM E code chapter are located either in Chapter 19: Injury, poisoning and certain other consequences of external causes, or Chapter 20: External causes of morbidity. Codes in Chapter 20 capture the cause of the injury or health condition, the intent (unintentional or accidental; or intentional, such as suicide or assault), the place where the event occurred, the activity of the patient at the time of the event, and the person's status (i.e., civilian, military).

---

*Example:*

ICD-9-CM      Supplementary Classification of External Causes of Injury and Poisoning (E800-E999)

ICD-10-CM      Chapter 20: External causes of morbidity (V00-Y99)

---

*Examples:*
- ➤ W21.03XA, Struck by baseball, initial encounter
- ➤ Y92.320, Baseball field as the place of occurrence of the external cause
- ➤ Y93.64, Activities involving other sports and athletics played as a team or group: baseball
- ➤ Y99.8, Other external cause status (recreation or sport not for income or while a student)

# Section 1 Review Questions

*musculoskeletal*

1.  Gout is classified to the ___C___ chapter in ICD-10-CM.
    a.  Certain infectious and parasitic diseases
    b.  Endocrine, nutritional and metabolic diseases
    c.  Musculoskeletal system and connective tissue
    d.  Symptoms, signs and abnormal clinical and laboratory findings, NEC

2.  True or false? The United States it the only industrialized nation that has not yet implemented ICD-10-CM.
    a.  True
    b.  False

3.  All of the following are structural differences between ICD-9-CM and ICD-10-CM, *except:*
    a.  Addition of a sixth character in some chapters
    b.  Addition of placeholder
    c.  Diseases and conditions of the eyes and ears are classified in the same chapter as diseases of the nervous system
    d.  Postoperative complications have been moved to procedure-specific body system chapters

4.  True or false? The WHO version of ICD-10 will be implemented in the United States in 2014.
    a.  True          ICD-10-CM
    b.  False

5.  Which of the following is a feature of ICD-10-CM?
    a.  Combination codes have been created for both symptom and diagnosis
    b.  The obstetric codes indicate which trimester the patient is in rather than episode of care
    c.  Codes for postoperative complications have been expanded and a distinction has been made between intraoperative complications and post-procedural disorders
    d.  All of the above

6.  Which of the following statements is true?
    a.  All codes in ICD-10-CM include full code titles
    b.  All chapters in ICD-10-CM require the addition of code extensions
    c.  All codes in ICD-10-CM are seven characters in length
    d.  All codes in ICD-10-CM use the placeholder X

7.  The ICD-10-CM code to report a disease of the genitourinary system begins with what letter?
    a.  P
    b.  G
    c.  E
    d.  N

8.  Which of the following is a true statement regarding ICD-10-CM codes?
    a.  No decimals are used.
    b.  The first character is always an alpha.
    c.  Consist of three to five characters.
    d.  The second and third characters are always numeric.

9.    Which of the following is a valid ICD-10-CM code?
      a.    428.9
      b.    L03.313
      c.    T37.0XX1A
      d.    M12X.58

10.   True or false? The GEMs are a crosswalk between ICD-9-CM and ICD-10-CM.
      a.    True
      b.    False

# Section 2 – ICD-10-CM Conventions and Coding Guidelines

## *ICD-10-CM Conventions*

Correct assignment of ICD-10-CM diagnosis codes is dependent upon the individual understanding certain conventions used in the classification system. Similar to ICD-9-CM, abbreviations, punctuation, symbols, and notes are used as conventions and have special meanings that affect code assignment.

### *Placeholder Character*

ICD-10-CM utilizes a placeholder which is always the letter X and it has two uses:
- As the fifth character for certain six character codes. The X provides for future expansion without disturbing the sixth character structure.

---

*Examples:*
- ➢ T37.0X1A, Poisoning by sulfonamides, accidental (unintentional), initial encounter
- ➢ T56.0X2S, Toxic effect of lead and its compounds, intentional self-harm, sequela

---

- When a code has less than six characters and a seventh character is required. The X is assigned for all characters less than six in order to meet the requirement of coding to the highest level of specificity.

---

*Examples:*
- ➢ W85.XXXA, Exposure to electric transmission lines, initial encounter
- ➢ S17.0XXA, Crushing injury of larynx and trachea. initial encounter
- ➢ S01.02XA, Laceration with foreign body of scalp, initial encounter

---

### *Seventh Characters*

Some ICD-10-CM categories require a seventh character to provide further specificity about the condition being coded. This seventh character may be a number or letter and must always be the seventh character.

---

*Examples:*
- ➢ O65.0XX1, Obstructed labor due to deformed pelvis, fetus 1
- ➢ S02.110B, Type I occipital condyle fracture, initial encounter for open fracture
- ➢ T17.220D, Food in pharynx causing asphyxiation, subsequent encounter

---

**Activity – Placeholders and Seventh Characters**
To gain a greater understanding of the purpose of the X placeholder and the seventh character, refer to the Tabular List, locate the following, and determine the use of
- The seventh character for subcategory codes R40.21, R40.22, and R40.23
- The seventh character for category M80
- The X placeholder in subcategory O45.8
- The X placeholder in category X78

## Abbreviations

Not Elsewhere Classified (NEC) – ICD-10-CM, like its predecessors, contains codes to classify any and all conditions. A residual category, subdivision, or subclassification provides a location for "other" types of specified conditions that have not been classified anywhere else in the code set. These residual codes may also contain the term "NEC" as part of their descriptor. The Alphabetic Index uses NEC for a code description that will direct the coder to the Tabular List showing an Other Specified code description.

> *Example:*
> | *ICD-10-CM* | *ICD-9-CM* |
> |---|---|
> | H26.8  Other specified cataract | 366.8  Other cataract |
> | I25.89 Other forms of chronic ischemic heart disease | 414.8  Other specified forms of chronic ischemic heart disease |

Not Otherwise Specified (NOS) – The unspecified or Not Otherwise Specified (NOS) codes are available for use when the documentation of the condition identified by the provider is insufficient to assign a more specific code.

> *Example:*
> | *ICD-10-CM* | *ICD-9-CM* |
> |---|---|
> | H40.9  Unspecified glaucoma | 365.9  Unspecified glaucoma |
> | J12.9  Viral pneumonia, unspecified | 480.9  Viral pneumonia, unspecified |

## Punctuation

Similar to ICD-9-CM, punctuation is used in both the Alphabetic Index and the Tabular List. The types of punctuation included in ICD-10-CM are parentheses, brackets, and colons.

( ) Parentheses – Parentheses are used in both the Alphabetic Index and the Tabular List to enclose supplementary words that may be present or absent in the statement of a disease without affecting the code number to which it is assigned. The terms within the parentheses are referred to as *nonessential modifiers*.

> *Examples:* Alphabetic Index
> - **Anemia** (essential) (general) (hemoglobin deficiency) (infantile) (primary) (profound)
> - **Diabetes, diabetic** (mellitus) (sugar)
> - **Hemophilia** (classical) (familial) (hereditary)

> *Examples:* Tabular List
> - H44.611, Retained (old) magnetic foreign body in anterior chamber, right eye
> - I10, Essential (primary) hypertension
> - K51.011, Ulcerative (chronic) pancolitis with rectal bleeding

[ ] Brackets – The Tabular List uses square brackets to enclose synonyms, alternative wordings, or explanatory phrases. Brackets are used in the Alphabetic Index to identify manifestation codes.

---

*Examples:* Tabular List
  ➢ B06, Rubella [German measles]
  ➢ J00, Acute nasopharyngitis [common cold]

---

*Examples:* Alphabetic Index
  ☐ **Disease**, Alzheimer's G30.9 [F02.80]
  ☐ **Nephrosis**, in amyloidosis E85.4 [N08]

---

: Colon – Colons are used in the Tabular List after an incomplete term which needs one or more of the modifiers following the colon to make it assignable to a given category. The colon is used with both "includes" and "excludes" notes, in which the words that precede the colon are not considered complete terms and therefore must be appended by one of the modifiers indented under the statement before the condition can be assigned the correct code.

---

*Example:*
**G73.7 Myopathy in diseases classified elsewhere**
  *Excludes1:* myopathy in:
                rheumatoid arthritis (M05.32)
                sarcoidosis (D86.87)
                scleroderma (M34.82)
                sicca syndrome [Sjögren] (M35.03)
                systemic lupus erythematosus (M32.19)

---

**Note:** Other ICD-10-CM format issues that are different from ICD-9-CM to make note of:
  • Some symbols, that is, the lozenge, section mark, and braces are not included in ICD-10-CM.
  • Dashes are used in both the ICD-10-CM Alphabetic Indexes and the Tabular List.
    ○ The indexes utilize the dash at the end of a code number to indicate the code is incomplete. To determine the additional character(s), locate the code in the Tabular List, review the options, and assign the appropriate code.

      ▪ **Fracture, pathologic**
        ankle M84.47-
        carpus M84.44-
    ○ In the Tabular List, a dash preceded by a decimal point (.-) indicates an incomplete code. To determine the additional characters, locate the referenced category or subcategory elsewhere in the Tabular List, review the options, and assign the appropriate code.
      ▪ **J43 Emphysema**
        *Excludes1:* emphysematous (obstructive) bronchitis (J44.-)

---

### *Instructional Notes*

Similar to ICD-9-CM a variety of notes appear in both the Alphabetic Index and Tabular List of ICD-10-CM. The various types of notes are "includes" and "excludes" notes, "code first" notes, "use additional code" notes, and cross reference notes.

Inclusion Notes – Includes notes are used as conventions in the ICD-10-CM Tabular List to clarify the conditions included within a particular chapter, section, category, subcategory, or code. It is important to remember that the list of inclusions terms is not exhaustive and may include diagnoses not listed in the inclusion note. Inclusion notes are introduced by the word "includes" when appearing at the beginning of a chapter, section, or category.

---

*Example:*

**K25    Gastric Ulcer**
    *Includes:* erosion (acute) of stomach
                 pylorus ulcer (peptic)
                 stomach ulcer (peptic)

---

At the code level, the word "includes" does not precede the list of terms included in the code.

---

*Example:*

**K31.5  Obstruction of duodenum**
    Constriction of duodenum
    Duodenal ileus (chronic)
    Stenosis of duodenum
    Stricture of duodenum
    Volvulus of duodenum

---

Exclusion Notes – ICD-9-CM contains a single type of excludes note which has two different meanings leaving it to the coding professional to determine the correct meaning of the excludes note. In ICD-10-CM there are two types of excludes notes designated either as *Excludes1* or *Excludes2* in their title. Either or both may appear under a category, subcategory, or code.

The *Excludes1* note is a pure "excludes" note. It means *not coded here.* An *Excludes1* note indicates that the code excluded should never be used at the same time as the code above the *Excludes1* note. This note is used when two conditions cannot occur together, such as a congenital form versus an acquired form of the same condition.

---

*Example:*

**K51.4  Inflammatory polyps of colon**
    *Excludes1*: adenomatous polyp of colon (D12.6)
              polyposis of colon (D12.6)
              polyps of colon NOS (K63.5)

---

The *Excludes2* note means *not included here.* This type of "excludes" note indicates that the condition excluded is not part of the condition represented by the code, but a patient may have both conditions at the same time. When an *Excludes2* note appears under a code, it is acceptable to use both the code and the excluded code together if the patient has both conditions.

---

*Example:*

**J37.1  Chronic laryngotracheitis**
    *Excludes2*: acute laryngotracheitis (J04.2)
             acute tracheitis (J04.1)

---

Code First and Use Additional Code Notes – "Code first" and "use additional code" notes are similar to their counterparts in ICD-9-CM. Certain conditions have both an underlying etiology and multiple body system manifestations due to the underlying etiology. For such conditions, ICD-10-CM, similar to ICD-9-CM, has a coding convention that requires the underlying condition be sequenced first followed by the manifestation. The "use additional code" note appears at the etiology code and a "code first" note at the manifestation code.

---

*Example:*

**G30    Alzheimer's disease**
Use additional code to identify:
> dementia with behavioral disturbance (F02.81)
> dementia without behavioral disturbance (F02.80)

**F02    Dementia in other diseases classified elsewhere**
Code first the underlying physiological condition, such as
> Alzheimer's (G30.-)

**F02.80 Dementia in other diseases classified elsewhere, without behavioral disturbance**

**F02.81 Dementia in other diseases classified elsewhere, with behavioral disturbance**

---

Cross Reference Notes – Cross reference notes are used in the ICD-10-CM Alphabetic Index to advise the coding professional to look elsewhere before assigning a code. The three cross reference notes (*see, see also,* and *see condition*) are the same as those found in ICD-9-CM.

---

*Examples:*

**Pyocele**
- mastoid – *see* Mastoiditis, acute
- sinus (accessory) – *see* Sinusitis
- turbinate (bone) J32.9
- urethra (*see also* Urethritis) N34.0

**Mercurial** – *see condition*

**Mercurialism** – *see* subcategory T56.1

**Labyrinthitis** (circumscribed) (destructive) (diffuse) (inner ear) (latent) (purulent) (suppurative) – *see also* subcategory H83.0

---

---

**Activity 1 – Excludes Notes**
Explain, in common terms, the complete meaning of this code description and its notations.

**F06.1  Catatonic disorder due to known physiological condition**
  *Excludes1*:    catatonic stupor (R40.1)
             stupor NOS (R40.1)
  *Excludes2*:    catatonic schizophrenia (F20.2)
             dissociative stupor (F44.2)

**Activity 2 – Tabular Conventions**
To gain skills in identifying the different types of notes, open the Tabular List and review the following, comparing the ICD-10-CM entries to the ICD-9-CM entries for the same terms. Identify their similarities and differences.

- Find the note for C25.4, Malignant neoplasms of endocrine pancreas, and compare it to the note found under code 157.4 in ICD-9-CM.
- Locate the note for subcategory H62.4, Otitis externa in other diseases classified elsewhere, and review it against the note found under codes 380.13 and 380.15 in ICD-9-CM.
- Find the note for category J44, Other chronic obstructive pulmonary disease, and compare it to the note found under code 496 in ICD-9-CM.
- Locate the note for code O94, Sequelae of complication of pregnancy, childbirth and the puerperium, and determine how it is similar to the note found under code 677 in ICD-9-CM.

---

### Relational Terms

And – The term "and" is interpreted to mean "and/or" when it appears in a code title within the ICD-10-CM Tabular List.

With – The word "with" should be interpreted to mean "associated with" or "due to" when it appears in a code title, the Alphabetic Index, or an instructional note in the Tabular List. The term "with" in the Alphabetic Index is sequenced immediately following the main term, not in alphabetic order.

## ICD-10-CM Guidelines

In 2013 the National Center for Health Statistics (NCHS) revised the draft *ICD-10-CM Official Guidelines for Coding and Reporting.* These guidelines have been approved by the four organizations referred to as the Cooperating Parties for ICD-10-CM: the American Hospital Association (AHA), the American Health Information Management Association (AHIMA), the Centers for Medicare and Medicaid Services (CMS), and NCHS. The guidelines are organized into four sections similar to the *ICD-9-CM Official Guidelines for Coding and Reporting.* Section I includes the structure and conventions of the classification and general guidelines that apply to the entire classification in addition to chapter-specific guidelines that correspond to the chapters as they are arranged in the classification. Section II includes guidelines for selection of principal diagnosis for non-outpatient settings. Section III includes guidelines for reporting additional diagnoses in non-outpatient settings. Section IV is for outpatient coding and reporting.

The General Coding Guidelines (Part B of Section I) for ICD-10-CM are similar to their ICD-9-CM General Coding Guidelines counterparts with one additional guideline – Laterality. The Laterality Guideline states, "Some ICD-10-CM codes indicate laterality, specifying whether the condition occurs on the left, right or is bilateral. If no bilateral code is provided and the condition is bilateral, assign separate codes for both the left and right side. If the side is not identified in the medical record, assign the code for the unspecified side."

The complete 2013 version of the ICD-10-CM guidelines can be located on the NCHS website (http://www.cdc.gov/nchs/icd/icd10cm.htm).

**Activity – General Coding Guidelines**
To gain an understanding of the ICD-10-CM General Coding Guidelines, open the ICD-10-CM Official Guidelines (http://www.cdc.gov/nchs/icd/icd10cm.htm). Study Section I.B (pages 12–16).

The General Coding Guidelines for ICD-10-CM are similar to their ICD-9-CM General Coding Guidelines counterparts with a few exceptions, which are called out here:

- The Laterality (#13) Guideline states, "Some ICD-10-CM codes indicate laterality, specifying whether the condition occurs on the left, right or is bilateral. If no bilateral code is provided and the condition is bilateral, assign separate codes for both the left and right side. If the side is not identified in the medical record, assign the code for the unspecified side."
- Review the Documentation of Complications of Care (#16) Guidelines which states that "Code assignment is based on the provider's documentation of the relationship between the condition and the care or procedure." The guideline extends to any complications of care, regardless of the chapter the code is located in. It is important to note that not all conditions that occur during or following medical care or surgery are classified as complications. There must be a cause-and-effect relationship between the care provided and the condition and an indication in the documentation that it is a complication. If the complication is not clearly documented, query the provider for clarification.

# Section 2 Review Questions

1.   What is the purpose of the X in subcategory O45.8?
     a.   Describes laterality
     b.   To preserve the meaning of the sixth character
     c.   To provide further specificity about the condition being coded
     d.   To code to the highest level of specificity

2.   Which of the following abbreviations is used in ICD-10-CM?
     a.   NOC
     b.   NES
     c.   NEC
     d.   NIC

3.   True or false? ICD-10-CM uses inclusion terms in the same way that ICD-9-CM does.
     a.   True
     b.   False

4.   What indicates synonyms, alternative wording, or explanatory phrases in the Tabular List?
     a.   Parentheses
     b.   Brackets
     c.   Dash
     d.   Colon

5.   True or false? The seventh character is always a letter.
     a.   True
     b.   False

6.   True or false? ICD-10-CM contains codes that specify laterality.
     a.   True
     b.   False

7.   Which type of note is located under code H62.4?
     a.   Use additional code for manifestation
     b.   Code also external cause
     c.   Code first underlying disease
     d.   Includes

8.   Which of the following is a convention found in the Alphabetic Index of ICD-10-CM?
     a.   The colon
     b.   The abbreviation NEC
     c.   Use additional code notation
     d.   Code first notation

9.   True or false? For every code where ICD-10-CM provides codes for laterality, bilateral is listed as an option.
     a.   True
     b.   False

10.  True or false? Similar to ICD-9-CM, the term "with" is sequenced immediately following the main term.
     a.   True
     b.   False

## Section 3 – Organization and Classification of Diseases and Disorders – Chapters 1–7

This section is designed to present an overview of the changes to specific disorders and conditions classified to Chapters 1–7 of ICD-10-CM. Not every revision has been identified but certain conditions have been selected to point out concepts that represent organizational, terminology, and classification modifications.

### *Chapter 1: Certain infectious and parasitic diseases (A00-B99)*

Chapter 1 of ICD-10-CM includes categories A00-B99 arranged in the following blocks:

| | |
|---|---|
| A00-A09 | Intestinal infectious diseases |
| A15-A19 | Tuberculosis |
| A20-A28 | Certain zoonotic bacterial diseases |
| A30-A49 | Other bacterial diseases |
| A50-A64 | Infections with a predominantly sexual mode of transmission |
| A65-A69 | Other spirochetal diseases |
| A70-A74 | Other diseases caused by chlamydia |
| A75-A79 | Rickettsioses |
| A80-A89 | Viral and prion infections of the central nervous system |
| A90-A99 | Arthropod-borne viral fevers and viral hemorrhagic fevers |
| B00-B09 | Viral infections characterized by skin and mucous membrane lesions |
| B10 | Other human herpes viruses |
| B15-B19 | Viral hepatitis |
| B20 | Human immunodeficiency virus [HIV] disease |
| B25-B34 | Other viral diseases |
| B35-B49 | Mycoses |
| B50-B64 | Protozoal diseases |
| B65-B83 | Helminthiases |
| B85-B89 | Pediculosis, acariasis and other infestations |
| B90-B94 | Sequelae of infectious and parasitic diseases |
| B95-B97 | Bacterial and viral infectious agents |
| B99 | Other infectious diseases |

While overall Chapter 1 of ICD-10-CM is organized similar to ICD-9-CM, some category and subcategory titles have been changed.

| | | |
|---|---|---|
| *Examples:* | | |
| ICD-9-CM | 008, Intestinal infections due to other organisms | |
| ICD-10-CM | A08, Viral and other specified intestinal infections | |
| | | |
| ICD-9-CM | 024, Glanders | |
| ICD-9-CM | 025, Melioidosis | |
| ICD-10-CM | A24, Glanders and melioidosis | |
| | | |
| ICD-9-CM | 036.4, Meningococcal carditis | |
| ICD-10-CM | A39.5, Meningococcal heart disease | |

Certain diseases have also been rearranged in Chapter 1 of ICD-10-CM. For example, a separate subchapter, or block, has been created and appropriate conditions grouped together for Infections with a predominantly sexual mode of transmission (A50-A64). Two additional examples of separate blocks being created with the appropriate conditions grouped together are Viral hepatitis (B15-B19) and Other viral diseases (B25-B34).

Some terminology changes and revisions to the classification of specific infectious and parasitic disease in ICD-10-CM have occurred as well. For instance, the term *sepsis* has replaced *septicemia* throughout Chapter 1. Additionally, *streptococcal sore throat* and its inclusion terms found in the Infectious and Parasitic Disease chapter of ICD-9-CM are reclassified in ICD-10-CM to Chapter 10: Diseases of the respiratory system.

Many of the codes in Chapter 1 of ICD-10-CM have been expanded to reflect manifestations of the disease with the use of fourth or fifth characters allowing the infectious disease and manifestation to be captured in one code instead of two.

---

*Example:*
**A01.0  Typhoid fever**
Infection due to Salmonella typhi
A01.00, Typhoid fever, unspecified
A01.01, Typhoid meningitis
A01.02, Typhoid fever with heart involvement
A01.03, Typhoid pneumonia
A01.04, Typhoid arthritis
A01.05, Typhoid osteomyelitis
A01.09, Typhoid fever with other complications

---

**Activity – Chapter 1 Organization and Classification**
To learn more about these changes to the organization, terminology, and classification of infectious and parasitic diseases in ICD-10-CM, open the Tabular List. Review and compare the following entries and identify their differences. You will need access to the ICD-9-CM Tabular List to complete this review.

| ICD-10-CM | ICD-9-CM |
|---|---|
| B95-B97 | 041 |
| B94.1 | 139.0 |
| A48.1 | 482.84 |

---

## *Chapter 2: Neoplasms (C00-D49)*

Chapter 2 of ICD-10-CM includes categories C00-D49 arranged in the following blocks:

C00-C75     Malignant neoplasms stated or presumed to be primary (of specific sites) and certain specified histologies, except neuroendocrine, and of lymphoid, hematopoietic and related tissues

| | | |
|---|---|---|
| | C00-C14 | Malignant neoplasms of lip, oral cavity and pharynx |
| | C15-C26 | Malignant neoplasms of digestive organs |
| | C30-C39 | Malignant neoplasms of respiratory and intrathoracic organs |
| | C40-C41 | Malignant neoplasms of bone and articular cartilage |
| | C43-C44 | Malignant neoplasms of skin |
| | C45-C49 | Malignant neoplasms mesothelial and soft tissue |
| | C50 | Malignant neoplasms of breast |
| | C51-C58 | Malignant neoplasms of female genital organs |
| | C60-C63 | Malignant neoplasms of male genital organs |
| | C64-C68 | Malignant neoplasms of urinary tract |
| | C69-C72 | Malignant neoplasms of eye, brain and other parts of central nervous system |
| | C73-C75 | Malignant neoplasms of thyroid and other endocrine glands |
| C7A | | Malignant neuroendocrine tumors |
| C7B | | Secondary neuroendocrine tumors |
| C76-C80 | | Malignant neoplasms of ill-defined, other secondary and unspecified sites |
| C81-C96 | | Malignant neoplasm of lymphoid, hematopoietic and related tissue |
| D00-D09 | | In situ neoplasms |
| D10-D36 | | Benign neoplasms except benign neuroendocrine tumors |
| D3A | | Benign neuroendocrine tumors |
| D37-D48 | | Neoplasms of uncertain behavior, polycythemia vera and myelodysplastic syndromes |
| D49 | | Neoplasms of unspecified behavior |

The neoplasm chapter has undergone some organizational changes, too. For example, in ICD-10-CM, the block of codes for *in situ neoplasms* is located before the block for *benign neoplasms*. An example of a classification improvement is the addition in ICD-10-CM of a separate fifth character for extranodal and solid organ sites for lymphomas and Hodgkin's. ICD-9-CM included these sites with the fifth digit for unspecified site in codes for Hodgkin's disease, non-Hodgkin's lymphoma, peripheral, and cutaneous T-cell lymphomas.

---

**Activity – Chapter 2 Organization and Classification**

In order to gain a better understanding of modifications to the organization, terminology, and classification of neoplasms in ICD-10-CM, open the Tabular List. Locate the following categories and compare the presentation of the codes in ICD-10-CM to the codes in ICD-9-CM.

| ICD-10-CM | ICD-9-CM |
|---|---|
| C48 | 158 |
| C54 | 182 |
| C64-C68 | 189 |
| C80 | 199 |

---

# Chapter 3: Diseases of the blood and blood-forming organs and certain disorders involving the immune mechanism (D50-D89)

Chapter 3 of ICD-10-CM includes categories D50-D89 arranged in the following blocks:

| | |
|---|---|
| D50-D53 | Nutritional anemias |
| D55-D59 | Hemolytic anemias |
| D60-D64 | Aplastic and other anemias and other bone marrow failure syndromes |
| D65-D69 | Coagulation defects, purpura and other hemorrhagic conditions |
| D70-D77 | Other disorders of blood and blood-forming organs |
| D78 | Intraoperative and postprocedural complications of spleen |
| D80-D89 | Certain disorders involving the immune mechanism |

Coding professionals will find the organizational structure of ICD-10-CM's Chapter 3 an improvement over ICD-9-CM's Chapter 4, Diseases of the Blood and Blood-forming Organs. Diseases and disorders have been grouped into subchapters or blocks making it easier to identify the type of conditions classified to Chapter 3. Modifications have also been made to specific categories that bring the terminology up-to-date with current medical practice. Other enhancements to Chapter 3 include classification changes that provide greater specificity than found in ICD-9-CM.

---

*Example 1:*

| | | |
|---|---|---|
| ICD-9-CM | 281.2 | Folate-deficiency anemia |
| ICD-10-CM | D52 | Folate deficiency anemia |
| | | D52.0, Dietary folate deficiency anemia |
| | | D52.1, Drug-induced folate deficiency anemia |
| | | Code first (T36-T50) to identify drug |
| | | D52.8, Other folate deficiency anemias |
| | | D52.9, Folate deficiency anemia, unspecified |

---

*Example 2:*

| | | |
|---|---|---|
| ICD-9-CM | 282.4 | Thalassemias |
| ICD-10-CM | D56 | Thalassemia |
| | | D56.0, Alpha thalassemia |
| | | D56.1, Beta thalassemia |
| | | D56.2, Delta-beta thalassemia |
| | | D56.3, Thalassemia minor |
| | | D56.4, Hereditary persistence of fetal hemoglobin [HPFH] |
| | | D56.8, Other thalassemias |
| | | D56.9, Thalassemia, unspecified |

---

The last block in this chapter (D80-D89) groups disorders involving the immune mechanism. The immunodeficiency disorders have been reclassified from Chapter 4: Endocrine, Nutritional and Metabolic Diseases, and Immunity Disorders in ICD-9-CM to Chapter 3 in ICD-10-CM.

**Activity – Chapter 3 Organization and Classification**
To expand your knowledge of the alterations made to the organization, terminology, and classification of diseases of the blood and blood-forming organs and certain disorders involving the immune mechanism in ICD-10-CM, open the Tabular List. Find the following codes or categories and determine what changes were made between ICD revisions. You will need access to ICD-9-CM to complete this review.

| ICD-10-CM | ICD-9-CM |
|-----------|----------|
| D51.0 | 281.0 |
| D73 | 289 |
| D86 | 135 |

# Chapter 4: Endocrine, nutritional and metabolic diseases (E00-E89)

Chapter 4 of ICD-10-CM includes categories E00-E90 arranged in the following blocks:

| | |
|---|---|
| E00-E07 | Disorders of thyroid gland |
| E08-E13 | Diabetes mellitus |
| E15-E16 | Other disorders of glucose regulation and pancreatic internal secretion |
| E20-E35 | Disorders of other endocrine glands |
| E36 | Intraoperative complications of endocrine system |
| E40-E46 | Malnutrition |
| E50-E64 | Other nutritional deficiencies |
| E65-E68 | Overweight, obesity and other hyperalimentation |
| E70-E88 | Metabolic disorders |
| E89 | Postprocedural endocrine and metabolic complications and disorders, not elsewhere classified |

A number of new subchapters have been added to the chapter for endocrine, nutritional, and metabolic diseases. For example, diabetes mellitus and malnutrition have their own subchapter while these conditions were grouped with diseases of other endocrine glands and nutritional deficiencies respectively. Code titles have been revised in a number of places in Chapter 4.

**Note:** Code descriptors for goiter are now consistent with present terminology.

A significant change to ICD-10-CM is the classification of diabetes mellitus. Instead of a single category (250) as in ICD-9-CM, there are five categories for diabetes mellitus in ICD-10-CM. Additionally, diabetes mellitus codes have been expanded to reflect manifestations and complications of the disease by using fourth or fifth characters rather than by using an additional code to identify the manifestation. ICD-10-CM classifies inadequately controlled, out of control, and poorly controlled diabetes mellitus to diabetes mellitus, by type with hyperglycemia.

**Note:** ICD-10-CM's five categories for diabetes mellitus:
- E08, Diabetes mellitus due to underlying condition
- E09, Drug or chemical induced diabetes mellitus
- E10, Type 1 diabetes mellitus
- E11, Type 2 diabetes mellitus
- E13, Other specified diabetes mellitus

**Activity – Chapter 4 Organization and Classification**
To increase your understanding of the revisions to the organization, terminology, and classification of endocrine, nutritional, and metabolic diseases in ICD-10-CM, open the Tabular List. Next, ascertain the modifications by evaluating the ICD-9-CM information against what was found for the ICD-10-CM category or code. You will need access to ICD-9-CM to complete this review.

| ICD-10-CM | ICD-9-CM |
|---|---|
| E07.81 | 790.94 |
| E28.310-E28.319 | 256.31 |
| E32 | 254 |

## *Chapter 5: Mental, behavioral and neurodevelopmental disorders (F01-F99)*

As explained earlier, Chapter 5 contains more subchapters, categories, subcategories, and codes than ICD-9-CM. Rather than grouping by psychotic, nonpsychotic disorders, or mental retardation as in ICD-9-CM, ICD-10-CM organizes mental and behavioral disorders in the following blocks:

| | |
|---|---|
| F01-F09 | Mental disorders due to known physiological conditions |
| F10-F19 | Mental and behavioral disorders due to psychoactive substance use |
| F20-F29 | Schizophrenia, schizotypal, delusional, and other non-mood psychotic disorders |
| F30-F39 | Mood [affective] disorders |
| F40-F48 | Anxiety, dissociative, stress-related, somatoform and other nonpsychotic mental disorders |
| F50-F59 | Behavioral syndromes associated with physiological disturbances and physical factors |
| F60-F69 | Disorders of adult personality and behavior |
| F70-F79 | Intellectual disabilities |
| F80-F89 | Pervasive and specific developmental disorders |
| F90-F98 | Behavioral and emotional disorders with onset usually occurring in childhood and adolescence |
| F99 | Unspecified mental disorder |

Changes were necessary in many parts of Chapter 5 because of outdated terminology. For example, given what has been discovered in the past 20 years about the effects of nicotine, ICD-10-CM contains a separate category F17 for nicotine dependence with subcategories to identify the specific tobacco product and nicotine-induced disorders. ICD-9-CM has a single code, 305.1, for tobacco use disorder or tobacco dependence.

> **Note:** A fairly substantial classification change was made to the codes for drug and alcohol abuse and dependence

The identification of the stage of the substance use, namely continuous or episodic, is not a part of ICD-10-CM. A single ICD-10-CM code identifies not only the substance but also the disorder the substance use induced. There continues to be codes for substance dependence "in remission."

> **Coding Tip:** The codes in Chapter 5 of ICD-10-CM parallel the codes in DSM-IV TR in most cases.

> **Activity – Chapter 5 Organization and Classification**
> Refer to the Tabular List to find out more about the organization, terminology, and classification modifications to mental and behavioral disorders in ICD-10-CM. Locate the listed ICD-10-CM category or code. Then, evaluate the ICD-9-CM information against what was found and discern the variances.
>
> | *ICD-10-CM* | *ICD-9-CM* |
> |---|---|
> | F03 | 290.1 |
> | F10.1 | 305.0 |
> | F43.1 | 309.81 |

# Chapter 6: Diseases of the nervous system (G00-G99)

Chapter 6 of ICD-10-CM includes categories G00-G99 arranged in the following blocks:

| | |
|---|---|
| G00-G09 | Inflammatory diseases of the central nervous system |
| G10-G14 | Systemic atrophies primarily affecting the central nervous system |
| G20-G26 | Extrapyramidal and movement disorders |
| G30-G32 | Other degenerative diseases of the nervous system |
| G35-G37 | Demyelinating diseases of the central nervous system |
| G40-G47 | Episodic and paroxysmal disorders |
| G50-G59 | Nerve, nerve root and plexus disorders |
| G60-G65 | Polyneuropathies and other disorders of the peripheral nervous system |
| G70-G73 | Diseases of myoneural junction and muscle |
| G80-G83 | Cerebral palsy and other paralytic syndromes |
| G89-G99 | Other disorders of the nervous system |

The organization of Chapter 6 in ICD-10-CM is comparable to that in ICD-9-CM. One change to note is that only diseases of the nervous system are contained in Chapter 6 of ICD-10-CM. Diseases of the sense organs, namely eye/adnexa and ear/mastoid processes, each have their own chapter in ICD-10-CM while they are combined into a single chapter in ICD-9-CM. A few categories in Chapter 6 have rephrased titles and in some cases encompass a combination of conditions. Additionally, a number of codes for diseases of the nervous system have been expanded in ICD-10-CM.

---

**Note:**
- Category for Alzheimer's disease (G30) has been expanded to reflect onset (early versus late)
- ICD-10-CM has two codes for phantom limb syndrome, differentiating whether pain is present or not

---

**Note:** Classification of organic sleep disorders have undergone a significant change in ICD-10-CM:
- First, these disorders are now included in Chapter 6 rather than the signs and symptoms chapter where ICD-9-CM had classified them
- Second, sleep apnea has its own subcategory (G47.3) with fifth character specificity identifying the type

---

**Activity – Chapter 6 Organization and Classification**
To become more familiar with other revisions to the organization, terminology, and classification of diseases of the nervous system in ICD-10-CM, open the Tabular List. Find the ICD-10-CM category or code listed here and assess how it differs from the ICD-9-CM category or code.

| ICD-10-CM | ICD-9-CM |
|---|---|
| G01 | 320.7 |
| G40 | 345 |
| G43 | 346 |

## *Chapter 7: Diseases of eyes and adnexa (H00-H59)*

Chapter 7 of ICD-10-CM includes categories H00-H59 arranged in the following blocks:

| | |
|---|---|
| H00-H05 | Disorders of eyelid, lacrimal system and orbit |
| H10-H11 | Disorders of conjunctiva |
| H15-H22 | Disorders of sclera, cornea, iris and ciliary body |
| H25-H28 | Disorders of lens |
| H30-H36 | Disorders of choroid and retina |
| H40-H42 | Glaucoma |
| H43-H44 | Disorders of vitreous body and globe |
| H46-H47 | Disorders of optic nerve and visual pathways |
| H49-H52 | Disorders of ocular muscles, binocular movement, accommodation and refraction |
| H53-H54 | Visual disturbances and blindness |
| H55-H57 | Other disorders of eye and adnexa |
| H59 | Intraoperative and postprocedural complications and disorders of eye and adnexa, not elsewhere classified |

Chapter 7 is an entirely new chapter in ICD-10-CM. In ICD-9-CM, the conditions classified in this chapter are located in Chapter 6: Diseases of the Nervous System and Sense Organs. Chapter 7 in ICD-10-CM also has a different organization than what is found in ICD-9-CM. While the structure is still by "site" for diseases of the eye and adnexa, the order differs.

Some categories in Chapter 7 have undergone title changes to reflect the terminology used today. For example, ICD-9-CM uses *senile cataract* while ICD-10-CM utilizes the descriptor *age-related cataract*. Many of the classification changes in Chapter 7 have to do with the expansion of characters to provide for laterality. ICD-10-CM contains codes for right side, left side, and in some instances bilateral sides for diseases of the eye and adnexa.

---

*Example:*
**H16.01 Central corneal ulcer**
> H16.011, Central corneal ulcer, right eye
> H16.012, Central corneal ulcer, left eye
> H16.013, Central corneal ulcer, bilateral
> H16.019, Central corneal ulcer, unspecified eye

---

**Activity – Chapter 7 Organization and Classification**
For additional practice with learning the organization, terminology, and classification changes to the chapter of diseases of eyes and adnexa in ICD-10-CM, open the Tabular List. Review the ICD-10-CM category or code listed below and ascertain the modification.

| *ICD-10-CM* | *ICD-9-CM* |
|---|---|
| H02.6 | 374.51 |
| H40 | 365 |
| H49 | 378.50 |

# Section 4 – Chapters 1–7 Guidelines

This section is designed to highlight the revisions to the guidelines found in Chapters 1–7 of ICD-10-CM. All modifications have not been identified, but certain guiding principles have been selected to illustrate guideline variations from ICD-9-CM. Also included in this section is the review of chapter-specific coding guidelines published by NCHS.

## *Chapter 1: Certain infectious and parasitic diseases (A00-B99)*

At the beginning of Chapter 1 is an instruction to use an additional code to identify resistance to antimicrobial drugs (Z16). This new guideline should be followed when assigning any code from this chapter.

Guidelines for code usage may also be category specific.

> **Note:** Under ICD-10-CM category B39, histoplasmosis, is a note to use an additional code for any associated manifestation. This differs from the note in ICD-9-CM in that the manifestation would be coded using a fifth-digit classification.

The NCHS has published chapter-specific guidelines for Chapter 1 of ICD-10-CM:
- Guideline I.C.1.a. Human immunodeficiency virus [HIV] infections
- Guideline I.C.1.b. Infectious agents as the cause of diseases classified to other chapters
- Guideline I.C.1.c. Infections resistant to antibiotics
- Guideline I.C.1.d. Sepsis, severe sepsis, and septic shock

> **Activity – Chapter 1 Guidelines**
> To gain an understanding of these rules, access the 2013 guidelines from the NCHS website (http://www.cdc.gov/nchs/icd/icd10cm.htm) and read Chapter 1: Certain infectious and parasitic diseases guidelines, I.C.1.a through I.C.1.e.1.d on pages 16–24.

## *Chapter 2: Neoplasms (C00-D49)*

The NCHS has published chapter-specific guidelines for Chapter 2 of ICD-10-CM. Most of these guidelines are consistent with what we see in ICD-9-CM with a few exceptions. One guideline to take note of is I.C.2.c.1, Anemia associated with malignancy. This guideline states the following:

> When admission/encounter is for management of an anemia associated with the malignancy, and the treatment is only for anemia, the appropriate code for the malignancy is sequenced as the principal or first-listed diagnosis followed by the appropriate code for the anemia (such as code D63.0, Anemia in neoplastic disease).

The appropriate sequencing can be easily confused with the next guideline (I.C.2.c.2) for Anemia associated with chemotherapy, immunotherapy and radiation therapy, which states:

> When the admission/encounter is for management of an anemia associated with an adverse effect of the administration of chemotherapy or immunotherapy and the only treatment is for the anemia, the anemia code is sequenced first followed by the appropriate codes for the neoplasm and the adverse effect (T45.1X5, Adverse effect of antineoplastic and immunosuppressive drugs).

When the admission/encounter is for management of an anemia associated with an adverse effect of radiotherapy, the anemia code should be sequenced first, followed by the appropriate neoplasm code and code Y84.2, Radiological procedure and radiotherapy as the cause of abnormal reaction of the patient, or of later complication, without mention of misadventure at the time of the procedure.

---

**Activity – Chapter 2 Guidelines**

To gain an understanding of these rules, access the 2013 guidelines from the NCHS website (http://www.cdc.gov/nchs/icd/icd10cm.htm) and read Chapter 2: Neoplasm guidelines, I.C.2.a through I.C.2.r on pages 24–31.

---

## Chapter 3: Diseases of the blood and blood-forming organs and certain disorders involving the immune mechanism (D50-D89)

At this time, there are no chapter-specific guidelines related to Chapter 3: Diseases of the blood and blood-forming organs and certain disorders involving the immune mechanism. There are important instructional notes throughout Chapter 3 that the coder should be aware of.

---

*Examples:*

**D61.2  Aplastic anemia due to other external agents**

Code first, if applicable, toxic effects of substances chiefly nonmedicinal as to source (T51-T65)

**D70.1  Agranulocytosis secondary to cancer chemotherapy**

Use additional code for adverse effect, if applicable, to identify drug (T45.1X5)

Code also underlying neoplasm

---

# Chapter 4: Endocrine, nutritional and metabolic diseases (E00-E89)

Instructions for coding "late effects" or sequelae have been expanded in Chapter 4 of ICD-10-CM. For example, *Excludes1* notes have been added to some categories between E50-E63 to indicate that the sequelae of the nutritional deficiency are assigned a code from category E64.

New guidelines that clarify code usage are also found under specific codes.

> **Note:** Under code E34.0, Carcinoid syndrome, is a note that states "May be used as an additional code to identify functional activity associated with a carcinoid tumor."
>
> No such note appears under the ICD-9-CM code 259.2 for this same condition.

The NCHS has published chapter-specific guidelines for Chapter 4 of ICD-10-CM:
- Guideline I.C.4.a. Diabetes mellitus

> **Activity – Chapter 4 Guidelines**
> To gain an understanding of these rules, access the 2013 guidelines from the NCHS website (http://www.cdc.gov/nchs/icd/icd10cm.htm) and read Chapter 4: Endocrine, nutritional and metabolic diseases guidelines I.C.4.a.1 through I.C.4.a.6 on pages 31–33.

# Chapter 5: Mental and behavioral disorders (F01-F99)

Many changes were made to Chapter 5, including organization and terminology, which resulted in some guideline adjustments as well.

> *Example* In ICD-10-CM beneath code F54, Psychological and behavioral factors associated with disorders or diseases classified elsewhere, there is a note that states to "code first the associated physical disorder."
>
> The equivalent ICD-9-CM code, 316, has a note to "use additional code to identify the associated physical condition."

The NCHS has published chapter-specific guidelines for Chapter 5 of ICD-10-CM. Take note of Guideline I.C.5.c.2, which describes the hierarchy rules for coding psychoactive substance use, abuse, and dependence.

> **Activity – Chapter 5 Guidelines**
> To gain an understanding of these rules, access the 2013 guidelines from the NCHS website (http://www.cdc.gov/nchs/icd/icd10cm.htm) and read Chapter 5: Mental, behavioral, and neurodevelopmental disorders guidelines I.C.5.a through I.C.5.c on pages 33–34.

## *Chapter 6: Diseases of the nervous system (G00-G99)*

In ICD-10-CM, there is a series of excluded conditions listed at the beginning of Chapter 6 that are applicable to all conditions within the nervous system chapter.

There are also additional guideline modifications made to specific codes.

*Example:* In ICD-10-CM beneath category G89, Pain, not elsewhere classified, there is a note that states "code also related psychological factors associated with pain."

However, below ICD-9-CM category 338, Pain, not elsewhere classified, the note instructs coding professionals to "use additional code to identify pain associated with psychological factors (307.89)."

The NCHS has published chapter-specific guidelines for Chapter 6 of ICD-10-CM that focus on dominant/nondominant side and pain.

**Activity – Chapter 6 Guidelines**
To gain an understanding of these rules, access the 2013 guidelines from the NCHS website (http://www.cdc.gov/nchs/icd/icd10cm.htm) and read Chapter 6: Diseases of the nervous system and sense organs guidelines I.C.6.a through I.C.6.b.6 on pages 34–38.

## *Chapter 7: Diseases of the eye and adnexa (H00-H59)*

With the formation of a new chapter for diseases of the eye and adnexa, come new instructions on which conditions are excluded from Chapter 7 of ICD-10-CM. Since the placement of the note is at the beginning of Chapter 7, none of the listed conditions would be coded here.

Included in this chapter are a number of guidelines for code usage that are code specific.

**Note:** Under ICD-10-CM subcategory H47.5, Disorders of other visual pathways, is a note to code also the underlying condition. This differs from ICD-9-CM in that a single code is used to identify the visual pathway disorder and the associated condition.

**Note:** Under ICD-10-CM subcategory H54, Blindness and low vision, is a note to code first any associated underlying cause of the blindness. No such note appears under ICD-9-CM category 369, Blindness and low vision.

**Activity – Chapter 7 Guidelines**
To gain an understanding of these rules, access the 2013 guidelines from the NCHS website (http://www.cdc.gov/nchs/icd/icd10cm.htm) and read Chapter 7: Diseases of the eye and adnexa guidelines I.C.7.a through I.C.7.a.5 on pages 38–39.

# Sections 3 and 4 Review Questions

1. True or false? In ICD-10-CM, code B20 is used to report a diagnosis of symptomatic HIV disease.
   a. True
   b. False

2. What is the correct code(s) for bilateral acute conjunctivitis, unspecified?
   a. H10.31, H10.32
   b. H10.33
   c. H10.233
   d. H10.13

3. True or false? Bacteremia and septicemia NOS are coded to R65.2.
   a. True
   b. False

4. What is the correct ICD-10-CM code(s) for premature menopause with sleeplessness?
   a. N95.1
   b. E28.3, G47.0
   c. E28.310
   d. E28.319

5. True or false? In ICD-10-CM, all diabetes mellitus codes require documentation of whether the condition is under control.
   a. True
   b. False

6. True or false? A malignant neoplasm code should not be assigned as principal diagnosis if the care involved surgical removal of the neoplasm along with adjunct chemotherapy during the same episode of care.
   a. True
   b. False

7. The fifth character for category G43, Migraine, denotes what?
   a. Intractable or not intractable
   b. With or without mention of seizures
   c. With or without aura
   d. With or without prolonged aura

8. True or false? ICD-10-CM provides for greater specificity of diseases of the spleen than ICD-9-CM.
   a. True
   b. False

9. In cases where the affected side is documented, but not specified as dominant or nondominant, how should right side monoplegia be classified?
   a. Dominant
   b. Nondominant
   c. Unspecified
   d. Undetermined

10. When an encounter is for pain management due to the malignancy, what code should be sequenced first?
    a. Primary malignancy or appropriate metastatic site code
    b. The pain code
    c. Encounter for cancer staging
    d. Observation for suspected neoplasm

# Section 5 – Organization and Classification of Diseases and Disorders – Chapters 8–14

This section is designed to present an overview of the changes to specific disorders classified to Chapters 8–14 of ICD-10-CM. Not every revision has been identified but certain conditions have been selected to point out concepts that represent organizational, terminology, and classification modifications.

## *Chapter 8: Diseases of the ear and mastoid process (H60-H95)*

Chapter 8 of ICD-10-CM includes categories H60-H95 arranged in the following blocks:

| | |
|---|---|
| H60-H62 | Diseases of external ear |
| H65-H75 | Diseases of middle ear and mastoid |
| H80-H83 | Diseases of inner ear |
| H90-H94 | Other disorders of ear |
| H95 | Intraoperative and postprocedural complications and disorders of ear and mastoid process, not elsewhere classified |

Chapter 8 is an entirely new chapter in ICD-10-CM. In ICD-9-CM, the conditions classified in this chapter are located in Chapter 6: Diseases of the Nervous System and Sense Organs. Diseases of the ear and mastoid process have been arranged into blocks making it easier to identify the types of conditions that would occur in the external ear (block 1), middle ear and mastoid (block 2), and inner ear (block 3). Block 4 is used for other disorders of the ear. Block 5 contains the codes for intraoperative and postprocedural complications. The intraoperative and postprocedural complications are grouped at the end of the chapter rather than scattered throughout different categories. Category and subcategory titles have been revised in a number of locations in Chapter 8.

---

*Examples:*

| | |
|---|---|
| ICD-9-CM | 381, Nonsuppurative otitis media and Eustachian tube disorders |
| ICD-10-CM | H65, Nonsuppurative otitis media |
| | |
| ICD-9-CM | 380.10, Infective otitis externa, unspecified |
| ICD-10-CM | H60.0, Abscess of external ear |
| | |
| ICD-9-CM | 386, Vertiginous syndromes and other disorders of vestibular system |
| ICD-10-CM | H81, Disorders of vestibular function |

---

Although Chapter 8 in ICD-10-CM basically parallels the corresponding section in Chapter 6 of ICD-9-CM, there are quite a few changes. These changes include greater specificity added at the fourth-, fifth-, and sixth-character levels; the delineation of laterality; and the addition of many more "code first underlying disease" notes.

One last noted classification change in this chapter is that the ICD-9-CM category 381, Nonsuppurative otitis media and Eustachian tube disorders, has been split into two categories in ICD-10-CM; H65, Nonsuppurative otitis media and H68, Eustachian salpingitis and obstruction.

**Activity – Chapter 8 Organization and Classification**
To expand your knowledge of the alterations made to the organization, terminology, and classification of diseases of the ear and mastoid, refer to the Tabular List of ICD-10-CM, find the following codes or categories, and identify what changes were made between ICD revisions.

| ICD-10-CM | ICD-9-CM |
|-----------|----------|
| H65 | 381 |
| H81.0 | 386.0 |
| H83.2 | 386.5 |

# Chapter 9: Diseases of the circulatory system (I00-I99)

Chapter 9 of ICD-10-CM includes categories I00-I99 arranged in the following blocks:

| | |
|---|---|
| I00-I02 | Acute rheumatic fever |
| I05-I09 | Chronic rheumatic heart diseases |
| I10-I15 | Hypertensive diseases |
| I20-I25 | Ischemic heart diseases |
| I26-I28 | Pulmonary heart disease and diseases of pulmonary circulation |
| I30-I52 | Other forms of heart disease |
| I60-I69 | Cerebrovascular diseases |
| I70-I79 | Diseases of arteries, arterioles and capillaries |
| I80-I89 | Diseases of veins, lymphatic vessels and lymph nodes, not elsewhere classified |
| I95-I99 | Other and unspecified disorders of the circulatory system |

The organization of Chapter 9 in ICD-10-CM is comparable to Chapter 7 in ICD-9-CM. One change to note is the order of conditions within the block for ischemic heart disease.

**Note:** In ICD-9-CM, the first condition is acute myocardial infarction. However, in ICD-10-CM angina pectoris begins the block for ischemic heart disease.

The terminology used to describe several cardiovascular conditions has been revised to reflect more current medical practice.

*Examples:*

| | |
|---|---|
| ICD-9-CM | 410, Acute myocardial infarction |
| ICD-10-CM | I21, ST elevation (STEMI) and non-ST elevation (NSTEMI) myocardial infarction |
| | |
| ICD-9-CM | 411.1, Intermediate coronary syndrome |
| ICD-10-CM | I20.0, Unstable angina |
| | |
| ICD-9-CM | 411.81, Acute coronary occlusion without myocardial infarction |
| ICD-10-CM | I24.0, Acute coronary thrombosis not resulting in myocardial infarction |

Some revisions to the classification have occurred as well.

**Note:** In ICD-9-CM, the code for gangrene (785.4) is classified in Chapter 16: Symptoms, Signs and Ill-Defined Conditions whereas in ICD-10-CM this condition is classified in Chapter 9 and is coded as I96, Gangrene, NEC. Additionally, Binswanger's disease has been reclassified from Chapter 5, Mental Disorders, in ICD-9-CM to Chapter 9 in ICD-10-CM and is coded as I67.3.

One last noted change is with the classification of hypertension. In ICD-9-CM, hypertension codes classify the type of hypertension (benign, malignant, unspecified). In ICD-10-CM, hypertension codes no longer classify the type.

**Activity – Chapter 9 Organization and Classification**
To learn more about these changes to the organization, terminology, and classification of diseases of the circulatory system refer to the ICD-10-CM Tabular List, review and compare the following entries, and identify their differences.

| ICD-10-CM | ICD-9-CM |
|---|---|
| I25.1 | 414.01 |
| I40.0, I40.1 | 422.91, 422.92 |
| I43 | 425.8 |

# *Chapter 10: Diseases of the respiratory system (J00-J99)*

Chapter 10 of ICD-10-CM includes categories J00-J99 arranged in the following blocks:

| | |
|---|---|
| J00-J06 | Acute upper respiratory infections |
| J09-J18 | Influenza and pneumonia |
| J20-J22 | Other acute lower respiratory infections |
| J30-J39 | Other diseases of upper respiratory tract |
| J40-J47 | Chronic lower respiratory diseases |
| J60-J70 | Lung diseases due to external agents |
| J80-J84 | Other respiratory diseases principally affecting the interstitium |
| J85-J86 | Suppurative and necrotic conditions of the lower respiratory tract |
| J90-J94 | Other diseases of the pleura |
| J95 | Intraoperative and postprocedural complications and disorders of respiratory system, not elsewhere classified |
| J96-J99 | Other diseases of the respiratory system |

While overall Chapter 10 of ICD-10-CM is organized similar to ICD-9-CM, diseases have been rearranged.

Modifications have also been made to specific categories that bring the terminology up-to-date with current medical practice.

---

**Note:**
- ICD-10-CM category J43, Emphysema, contains codes with panlobular emphysema and centrilobular emphysema in their titles
- ICD-10-CM category, J45, Asthma, classifies asthma as mild intermittent, mild persistent, moderate persistent, and severe persistent.

---

Other enhancements to Chapter 10 include classification changes that provide greater specificity than found in ICD-9-CM.

---

**Note:**
- ICD-10-CM has individual codes for acute recurrent sinusitis for each sinus whereas ICD-9-CM does not have a specific code for acute recurrent sinusitis
- ICD-10-CM subcategory J10.8, Influenza due to other identified influenza virus with other manifestations, has been expanded to reflect the manifestations of the influenza
- ICD-10-CM category J20, Acute bronchitis, has been expanded to reflect the manifestations of the acute bronchitis.

---

**Activity – Chapter 10 Organization and Classification**

To become more familiar with other revisions to the organization, terminology, and classification of diseases of the respiratory system refer to the ICD-10-CM Tabular List and find the ICD-10-CM category or code for those listed here. Assess how each differs from ICD-9-CM.

| *ICD-10-CM* | *ICD-9-CM* |
|---|---|
| J18.1 | 481 |
| J30-J39 | 470-478 |
| J45 | 493 |

## *Chapter 11: Diseases of the digestive system (K00-K95)*

Chapter 11 of ICD-10-CM includes categories K00-K95 arranged in the following blocks:

| | |
|---|---|
| K00-K14 | Diseases of oral cavity and salivary glands |
| K20-K31 | Diseases of esophagus, stomach and duodenum |
| K35-K38 | Diseases of appendix |
| K40-K46 | Hernia |
| K50-K52 | Noninfective enteritis and colitis |
| K55-K64 | Other diseases of intestines |
| K65-K68 | Diseases of peritoneum and retroperitoneum |
| K70-K77 | Diseases of liver |
| K80-K87 | Disorders of gallbladder, biliary tract and pancreas |
| K90-K95 | Other diseases of digestive system |

A number of new subchapters have been added to the chapter for diseases of the digestive system. For instance, in ICD-10-CM diseases of the liver have their own subchapter or block while these conditions were grouped with other diseases of the digestive system in ICD-9-CM. Some terminology changes and revisions to the classification of specific digestive conditions have occurred in ICD-10-CM as well.

---

**Note:** The term "hemorrhage" is used when referring to ulcers, and the term "bleeding" is used when classifying gastritis, duodenitis, diverticulosis, and diverticulitis
- K25.0, Acute gastric ulcer with hemorrhage
- K29.01, Acute gastritis with bleeding
- K57.31, Diverticulosis of large intestine without perforation or abscess with bleeding

---

ICD-10-CM category K50, Crohn's disease, has been expanded to the fourth, fifth, and sixth character in contrast to ICD-9-CM category 555, Regional enteritis. The expansion at the fourth character level specifies the site of the Crohn's disease, the fifth character indicates whether a complication was present, and the sixth character further classifies the specific complication.

In ICD-9-CM, the presence or absence of obstruction is used as an axis for classifying ulcers. In ICD-10-CM a fairly substantial classification change was made and the identification of obstruction is no longer a part of the ICD-10-CM ulcer code structure.

---

**Activity – Chapter 11 Organization and Classification**
To gain a better understanding of modifications to the organization, terminology, and classification of diseases of the digestive system, refer to the ICD-10-CM Tabular List, locate the following categories, and determine the revision.

| ICD-10-CM | ICD-9-CM |
|---|---|
| K22 | 530 |
| K37 | 541 |
| K62 | 569 |

---

# Chapter 12: Diseases of skin and subcutaneous tissue (L00-L99)

Chapter 12 of ICD-10-CM includes categories L00-L99 arranged in the following blocks:

| | |
|---|---|
| L00-L08 | Infections of the skin and subcutaneous tissue |
| L10-L14 | Bullous disorders |
| L20-L30 | Dermatitis and eczema |
| L40-L45 | Papulosquamous disorders |
| L49-L54 | Urticaria and erythema |
| L55-L59 | Radiation-related disorders of the skin and subcutaneous tissue |
| L60-L75 | Disorders of skin appendages |
| L76 | Intraoperative and postprocedural complications of skin and subcutaneous tissue |
| L80-L99 | Other disorders of the skin and subcutaneous tissue |

ICD-10-CM Chapter 12 represents a complete restructuring to bring together groups of diseases that are related to one another in some way. Additionally, greater specificity has been added to many of the codes at either the fourth-, fifth-, and even sixth-character level. ICD-9-CM Chapter 12 has only three subchapters which have been expanded in ICD-10-CM to create the nine blocks listed above.

One example of an organizational change to Chapter 12 of ICD-10-CM is a subchapter or block for ICD-10-CM codes for radiation-related disorders of the skin and subcutaneous tissue. The conditions found in this block are not located together in ICD-9-CM.

Some categories in Chapter 12 have undergone title changes to reflect terminology in use today. For instance, ICD-10-CM uses "androgenic alopecia" but this term is not used at all in ICD-9-CM.

An example of a classification improvement is the addition of characters in ICD-10-CM to represent the site and severity of the decubitus ulcer.

---

**Coding Tip:** While ICD-9-CM did add a subcategory for pressure ulcer stages in FY2009, two codes are required to code this specificity. ICD-10-CM provides the site (including laterality) and the stage all in one code.

---

**Activity – Chapter 12 Organization and Classification**
For additional practice with learning the organization, terminology, and classification changes to the chapter on diseases of skin and subcutaneous tissue, refer to the ICD-10-CM Tabular List and locate the following categories or codes. Ascertain the modifications.

| ICD-10-CM | ICD-9-CM |
|---|---|
| L03 | 681 |
| L03.32 | 682.2 |
| L98.4 | 707.1 |

## Chapter 13: Diseases of the musculoskeletal system and connective tissue (M00-M99)

Chapter 13 contains many more subchapters, categories, and codes than ICD-9-CM. Rather than having just four subchapters grouping many conditions together, ICD-10-CM organizes the musculoskeletal system and connective tissue in the following blocks:

| | |
|---|---|
| M00-M02 | Infectious arthropathies |
| M05-M14 | Inflammatory polyarthropathies |
| M15-M19 | Osteoarthritis |
| M20-M25 | Other joint disorders |
| M26-M27 | Dentofacial anomalies [including malocclusion] and other disorders of jaw |
| M30-M36 | Systemic connective tissue disorders |
| M40-M43 | Deforming dorsopathies |
| M45-M49 | Spondylopathies |
| M50-M54 | Other dorsopathies |
| M60-M63 | Disorders of muscles |
| M65-M67 | Disorders of synovium and tendon |
| M70-M79 | Other soft tissue disorders |
| M80-M85 | Disorders of bone density and structure |
| M86-M90 | Other osteopathies |
| M91-M94 | Chondropathies |
| M95 | Other disorders of the musculoskeletal system and connective tissue |
| M96 | Intraoperative and postprocedural complications and disorders of musculoskeletal system, not elsewhere classified |
| M99 | Biomechanical lesions, not elsewhere classified |

Almost every code in Chapter 13 of ICD-10-CM has been expanded in some way with the expansion including very specific sites as well as laterality. Numerous codes have been moved from various chapters in ICD-9-CM to Chapter 13 in ICD-10-CM.

---

*Examples:*

➤ Category 274, Gout in ICD-9-CM, Chapter 3: Endocrine, Nutritional and Metabolic Diseases and Immunity Disorders, is classified as M10, Gout, in ICD-10-CM Chapter 13

➤ Code 268.2, Osteomalacia, unspecified in ICD-9-CM Chapter 3 is classified to category M83, Adult osteomalacia in ICD-10-CM Chapter 13

➤ Code 524.4, Malocclusion, unspecified, in ICD-9-CM Chapter 9: Diseases of the Digestive System, is classified to code M26.4, Malocclusion, unspecified in ICD-10-CM Chapter 13

---

Category M80 in ICD-10-CM classifies the type of osteoporosis in addition to the site of a current pathological fracture into one combination code.

Additionally, some categories and subcategories in Chapter 13 require the use of seventh characters.

---

**Note:** The seventh characters are

| | |
|---|---|
| A | initial encounter for fracture |
| B | subsequent encounter for fracture with routine healing |
| G | subsequent encounter for fracture with delayed healing |
| K | subsequent encounter for fracture with nonunion |
| P | subsequent encounter for fracture with malunion |
| S | sequelae |

---

**Activity – Chapter 13 Organization and Classification**

To increase your understanding of the revisions to the organization, terminology, and classification of musculoskeletal system connective tissue diseases, refer to the ICD-10-CM Tabular List, locate the categories or codes listed below, and ascertain the modification by evaluating the ICD-9-CM information against the ICD-10-CM category or code.

| ICD-10-CM | ICD-9-CM |
|---|---|
| M10 | 274.9 |
| M15-M19 | 715 |
| M48.4 | 733.95 |

## *Chapter 14: Diseases of the genitourinary system (N00-N99)*

Chapter 14 of ICD-10-CM includes categories N00-N99 arranged in the following blocks:

| | |
|---|---|
| N00-N08 | Glomerular diseases |
| N10-N16 | Renal tubulo-interstitial diseases |
| N17-N19 | Acute kidney failure and chronic kidney disease |
| N20-N23 | Urolithiasis |
| N25-N29 | Other disorders of kidney and ureter |
| N30-N39 | Other diseases of the urinary system |
| N40-N53 | Diseases of male genital organs |
| N60-N65 | Disorders of breast |
| N70-N77 | Inflammatory diseases of female pelvic organs |
| N80-N98 | Noninflammatory disorders of female genital tract |
| N99 | Intraoperative and postprocedural complications and disorders of genitourinary system, not elsewhere classified |

For the most part, those genitourinary disorders in diseases classified elsewhere have been placed in their own category at the end of each block of Chapter 14. This differs from ICD-9-CM in that these conditions were classified within different subcategories.

**Note:** One category, N08, Glomerular disorders in diseases classified elsewhere, is used to identify glomerulonephritis, nephritis, and nephropathy in diseases classified elsewhere.

Changes were necessary in some sections of Chapter 14 because of outdated terminology. For example, given what has been discovered since the last revision of ICD about male erectile dysfunction, ICD-10-CM includes category N52 for this condition with subcategories to identify the different causes of the dysfunction. ICD-9-CM has a single code, 607.84, for impotence of organic origin.

**Coding Tip:** To code to the highest level of specificity for post-traumatic urethral stricture, coding professionals will need to identify the patient's gender. This is not necessary for ICD-9-CM code selection for this disorder.

**Activity – Chapter 14 Organization and Classification**
To find out more about the organization, terminology, and classification modifications to diseases of the genitourinary system, refer to the ICD-10-CM Tabular list and locate the ICD-10-CM category or code listed here. Then evaluate the ICD-9-CM information against what was found and discern the variances.

| *ICD-10-CM* | *ICD-9-CM* |
|---|---|
| N18 | 585 |
| N30 | 595 |
| N39.3 | 625.6/788.32 |

# Section 6 – Chapters 8–14 Guidelines

This section is designed to highlight the revisions to the guidelines found in Chapters 8–14 of ICD-10-CM. All modifications have not been illustrated but certain guiding principles have been selected to show guideline variations from ICD-9-CM. Also included in this section is the review of chapter-specific coding guidelines published by NCHS.

## *Chapter 8: Diseases of the ear and mastoid process (H60-H95)*

Guidelines on the use of codes may change from one revision to the next. For example, ICD-9-CM contains a note excluding otitis media with perforation of tympanic membrane from subcategory 384.2. In ICD-10-CM the note directly under H72, Perforation of tympanic membrane, states "code first any associated otitis media."

---

*Example:*

ICD-9-CM  **384.2, Perforation of Tympanic Membrane**
*Excludes*: otitis media with perforation of tympanic membrane (382.00-382.9)

ICD-10-CM  **H72, Perforation of tympanic membrane**
Code first any associated otitis media (H65.-, H66.1-, H66.2-, H66.3-, H66.4-, H66.9-,H67.-)
*Excludes1:* acute suppurative otitis media with rupture of the tympanic
         membrane (H66.01-)
         traumatic rupture of ear drum (S09.2-)

---

**Coding Tip:** There is an instructional note in categories H65, H66, and H67 to use an additional code for any associated perforated tympanic membrane (H72.-)

---

Another new guideline is found under the categories for nonsuppurative otitis media (H65) and suppurative and unspecified otitis media (H66). The note instructs coding professionals to use an additional code to identify: exposure to environmental tobacco smoke (Z77.22), exposure to tobacco smoke in the perinatal period (P96.81), history of tobacco use (Z87.891), occupational exposure to environmental tobacco smoke (Z57.31), tobacco dependence (F17.-), or tobacco use (Z72.0).

At this time, there are no chapter-specific guidelines related to Chapter 8: Diseases of the ears and mastoid process.

## *Chapter 9: Diseases of the circulatory system (I00-I99)*

There are guideline changes to a number of codes in this chapter. For example, in ICD-10-CM beneath categories I21, I22, and I23 for acute myocardial infarction are notes that state how the specific category must be used within four weeks (28 days) or less from onset. However, below category 410 in ICD-9-CM the note refers to an 8 week or less time period.

> **Note:** The instructional notes and guidelines are very important for these three categories to indicate correct code usage. A code from category I22, Subsequent acute myocardial infarction, must be used in conjunction with a code from category I21, ST elevation myocardial infarction (STEMI) and non-ST elevation myocardial infarction (NSTEMI). A code from category I23, certain current complications following ST elevation (STEMI) and non-ST elevation (NSTEMI) myocardial infarction must be used in conjunction with a code from category I21 or I22.

New guidelines that clarify code usage are also found under specific codes. Under code I05, rheumatic mitral valve diseases, is a note that states this category includes conditions classifiable to both I05.0 and I05.2-I05.9, whether specified as rheumatic or not.

The NCHS has published chapter-specific guidelines for Chapter 9 of ICD-10-CM:
- Guideline I.C.9.a. Hypertension
- Guideline I.C.9.b. Atherosclerotic coronary artery disease and angina
- Guideline I.C.9.c. Intraoperative and postprocedural cerebrovascular accident
- Guideline I.C.9.d. Sequelae of cerebrovascular disease
- Guideline I.C.9.e. Acute myocardial infarction

> **Activity – Chapter 9 Guidelines**
> To gain an understanding of these rules, access the 2013 guidelines from the NCHS website (http://www.cdc.gov/nchs/icd/icd10cm.htm) and read Chapter 9: Diseases of the circulatory system guidelines I.C.9.a through I.C.9.e.4 on pages 40–45.

## Chapter 10: Diseases of the respiratory system (J00-J99)

At the beginning of Chapter 10 the following instructional guideline appears: "When a respiratory condition is described as occurring in more than one site and is not specifically indexed, it should be classified to the lower anatomic site."

**Note:** Tracheobronchitis is classified to bronchitis in J40, Bronchitis, not specified as acute or chronic.

An additional instructional guideline also appears at the beginning of Chapter 10 which instructs the coding professional to use an additional code, where applicable to identify: exposure to environmental tobacco smoke (Z77.22), exposure to tobacco smoke in the perinatal period (P96.81), history of tobacco use (Z87.891), occupational exposure to environmental tobacco smoke (Z57.31), tobacco dependence (F17.-), or tobacco use (Z72.0).

**Coding Tip:** Since these new guidelines appear at the beginning of the chapter, they should be followed when assigning any code from this chapter.

Guidelines for code usage may also be category specific. Under ICD-10-CM category J10, influenza, is a note to use an additional code to identify the virus. No such note appears under the ICD-9-CM category (487) for this same condition.

The NCHS has published chapter-specific guidelines for Chapter 10 of ICD-10-CM:
- Guideline I.C.10.a. Chronic obstructive pulmonary disease and asthma
- Guideline I.C.10.b. Acute respiratory failure
- Guideline I.C.10.c. Influenza due to certain identified influenza viruses
- Guideline I.C.10.d. Ventilator-associated pneumonia

**Activity – Chapter 10 Guidelines**
To gain an understanding of these rules, access the 2013 guidelines from the NCHS website (http://www.cdc.gov/nchs/icd/icd10cm.htm) and read Chapter 10: Diseases of the respiratory system guidelines I.C.10.a through I.C.10.d.2 on pages 45–47.

## Chapter 11: Diseases of the digestive system (K00-K95)

Guideline modifications were made to specific codes in this chapter.

**Note:** For example, in ICD-9-CM ulcerative colitis does not have any instructions for code usage listed below category 556. In contrast, guidelines for category K51, Ulcerative colitis, state to use an additional code to identify manifestations.

No instructional note is found at the start of the subchapter for hernias in ICD-9-CM. However, this is not the case in ICD-10-CM. The note "Hernia with both gangrene and obstruction is classified to hernia with gangrene" applies to all conditions coded to categories K40–K46.

At this time, there are no chapter-specific guidelines related to Chapter 11: Diseases of the digestive system.

# Chapter 12: Diseases of the skin and subcutaneous tissue (L00-L99)

Instructions for coding dermatitis and eczema have been expanded in Chapter 12. For example, the note "In this block, the terms dermatitis and eczema are used synonymously and interchangeably" has been added to categories L20-L30. Additionally, the "excludes" note has been expanded in ICD-10-CM for categories L20-L30 compared to categories 690-698 in ICD-9-CM.

---

*Example:*

ICD-9-CM **Other Inflammatory Conditions of Skin and Subcutaneous Tissue (690-698)**
*Excludes*: panniculus (729.30-729.39)

ICD-10-CM **Dermatitis and Eczema (L20-L30)**
*Excludes2*:   chronic (childhood) granulomatous disease (D71)
dermatitis gangrenosa (L08.0)
dermatitis herpetiformis (L13.0)
dry skin dermatitis (L85.3)
factitial dermatitis (L98.1)
perioral dermatitis (L71.0)
radiation-related disorders of skin and subcutaneous
tissue (L55-L59)
stasis dermatitis (I83.1-I83.2)

---

The NCHS has published chapter-specific guidelines for Chapter 12 of ICD-10-CM:

- Guideline I.C.12.a. Pressure ulcer stage codes

**Activity – Chapter 12 Guidelines**
To gain an understanding of these rules, access the 2013 guidelines from the NCHS website (http://www.cdc.gov/nchs/icd/icd10cm.htm) and read Chapter 12: Diseases of the skin and subcutaneous tissue guidelines I.C.12.a.1 through I.C.12.a.6 on pages 47–48.

# Chapter 13: Diseases of the musculoskeletal system and connective tissue (M00-M99)

The first block of the chapter on diseases of the musculoskeletal system and connective tissue for infectious arthropathies includes arthropathies due to microbiological agents. To assist coding professionals on the correct usage of categories M00-M02, new guidelines provide definitions for direct and indirect infection.

---

**Coding Tip:** Distinction is made between the following types of etiological relationships:
- **Direct infection of joint**—where organisms invade synovial tissue and microbial antigen is present in the joint
- **Indirect infection**—which may be of two types: a reactive arthropathy, where microbial infection of the body is established but neither organisms nor antigens can be identified in the joint, and a postinfective arthropathy, where microbial antigen is present but recovery of an organism is inconstant and evidence of local multiplication is lacking

---

Instructional notes have also been added to different categories or subcategories to explain how codes should be assigned.

---

*Examples:*

**M21.7 Unequal limb length (acquired)**
Note: The site used should correspond to the shorter limb

**M50 Cervical disc disorders**
Note: Code to the most superior level of disorder

---

Notes have also been used to define terms.

---

*Examples:*

**M66 Spontaneous rupture of synovium and tendon**
Note: A spontaneous rupture is one that occurs when a normal force is applied to tissues that are inferred to have less than normal strength

**M80 Osteoporosis with current pathological fracture**
Note: Fragility fracture is defined as a fracture sustained with trauma no more than a fall from a standing height or less that occurs under circumstances that would not cause a fracture in a normal healthy bone

---

The NCHS has published chapter-specific guidelines for Chapter 13 of ICD-10-CM:
- Guideline I.C.13.a. Site and laterality
- Guideline I.C.13.b. Acute traumatic versus chronic or recurrent musculoskeletal conditions
- Guideline I.C.13.c. Coding of pathologic fractures
- Guideline I.C.13.d. Osteoporosis

---

**Activity – Chapter 13 Guidelines**
To gain an understanding of these rules, access the 2013 guidelines from the NCHS website (http://www.cdc.gov/nchs/icd/icd10cm.htm) and read Chapter 13: Diseases of the musculoskeletal system and connective tissue guidelines I.C.13.a through I.C.13.d.2 on pages 49–50.

---

## *Chapter 14: Diseases of the genitourinary system (N00-N99)*

Throughout Chapter 14 are new includes notes that help to clarify the types of disorders that are classified to the various categories.

---

*Example:*

**N00    Acute nephritis syndrome**

    *Includes*:    acute glomerular disease

                      acute glomerulonephritis

                      acute nephritis

**N71    Inflammatory disease of uterus, except cervix**

    *Includes*:    endo (myo) metritis

                      metritis

                      myometritis

                      pyometra

                      uterine abscess

---

A similar change has occurred to the instruction for menopausal and other perimenopausal disorders. In ICD-9-CM, there is no guideline under category 627 to help coding professionals in their selection of a code for these disorders. However, ICD-10-CM includes a note stating menopausal and other perimenopausal disorders due to naturally occurring (age-related) menopause and perimenopause are classified to category N95.

The NCHS has published chapter-specific guidelines for Chapter 14 of ICD-10-CM:

- Guideline I.C.14.a. Chronic kidney disease

---

**Activity – Chapter 14 Guidelines**

To gain an understanding of these rules, access the 2013 guidelines from the NCHS website (http://www.cdc.gov/nchs/icd/icd10cm.htm) and read Chapter 14: Diseases of the genitourinary system guidelines I.C.14.a.1 through I.C.14.a.3 on pages 50–51.

---

# Sections 5 and 6 Review Questions

1. True or false? If a patient with suppurative otitis media has a history of tobacco use, an additional code should be assigned.
   a. True
   b. False

2. According to NCHS Guidelines for Chapter 13 of ICD-10-CM, recurrent bone, joint, or muscle conditions are classified to which chapter?
   a. Chapter 13
   b. Chapter 18
   c. Chapter 19
   d. Chapter 20

3. True or false? The "code also" note found under ICD-10-CM category N17 should be interpreted to mean that the acute kidney failure should be assigned only as principal or first-listed.
   a. True
   b. False

4. True or false? If a patient has both acute systolic heart failure and hypertension, no causal condition relationship needs to be documented to use the combination code I11.0.
   a. True
   b. False

5. Review category I46. Which of the following is a false statement?
   a. Cardiac arrest is a non-specific principal diagnosis
   b. Code I46.8 is used as a secondary diagnosis code
   c. Code I46.2 is used as a secondary condition
   d. Cardiac arrest includes cardiogenic shock

6. True or false? The term "hemorrhage" is found in Chapter 11 in ICD-10-CM instead of the term "bleeding."
   a. True
   b. False

7. What is the correct ICD-10-CM code(s) for Crohn's disease of ileum with rectal bleeding and abscess?
   a. K50.011, K63.0
   b. K50.014
   c. K50.011, K50.014
   d. K50.014, K62.5

8. True or false? ICD-10-CM provides greater specificity than found in ICD-9-CM for acute recurrent sinusitis by providing an axis for recurrence.
   a. True
   b. False

9. Which of the following conditions is not classified to I40.1?
   a. Septic myocarditis
   b. Giant cell myocarditis
   c. Idiopathic myocarditis
   d. Fiedler's myocarditis

10.   The sixth character level for category L89 denotes what?
      a.    Site
      b.    Depth of the ulcer
      c.    Gangrene
      d.    Etiology

# Section 7 – Organization and Classification of Diseases and Disorders – Chapters 15–21

This section is designed to present an overview of the changes to specific disorders classified to Chapters 15–21 of ICD-10-CM. Not every revision has been identified but certain conditions have been selected to point out concepts that represent organizational, terminology, and classification modifications.

## Chapter 15: Pregnancy, childbirth and the puerperium (O00-O9A)

Chapter 15 of ICD-10-CM includes categories O00-O9A arranged in the following blocks:

| | |
|---|---|
| O00-O08 | Pregnancy with abortive outcome |
| O09 | Supervision of high risk pregnancy |
| O10-O16 | Edema, proteinuria and hypertensive disorders in pregnancy, childbirth and the puerperium |
| O20-O29 | Other maternal disorders predominantly related to pregnancy |
| O30-O48 | Maternal care related to the fetus and amniotic cavity and possible delivery problems |
| O60-O77 | Complications of labor and delivery |
| O80, O82 | Encounter for delivery |
| O85-O92 | Complications predominantly related to the puerperium |
| O94-O9A | Other obstetric conditions, not elsewhere classified |

With respect to classification changes, episode of care is no longer a secondary axis of classification for most conditions classified in Chapter 15. Instead ICD-10-CM identifies the trimester in which the condition occurred at the fifth- and sixth-character level.

Code titles have been revised in a number of locations in Chapter 15. For instance, ICD-9-CM's terminology states the indication for care such as inlet contractions of pelvis (653.2). ICD-10-CM terminology is much more descriptive of what the code represents, that is, maternal care for disproportion due to inlet contractions of pelvis (O33.2).

---

*Other Examples of Title Changes:*
ICD-9-CM      654, Abnormality of organs and soft tissues of pelvis
ICD-10-CM     O34, Maternal care for abnormality of pelvic organs

ICD-9-CM      664, Trauma to perineum and vulva during delivery
ICD-10-CM     O70, Perineal laceration during delivery

---

Codes for elective (legal or therapeutic) abortion are classified with the abortion codes in ICD-9-CM. In contrast, the elective abortion (without complication) code has been moved to code Z33.2, Encounter for elective termination of pregnancy, in Chapter 21 of ICD-10-CM. Complications of induced termination of pregnancy are found in category O04.

ICD-10-CM requires the use of a seventh character to identify the fetus to which certain complication codes apply.

---

*Example:*

**O32    Maternal care for malpresentation of fetus**

One of the following seventh characters is to be assigned to each code under category O32.

| | |
|---|---|
| 0 | not applicable or unspecified |
| 1 | fetus 1 |
| 2 | fetus 2 |
| 3 | fetus 3 |
| 4 | fetus 4 |
| 5 | fetus 5 |
| 9 | other fetus |

---

The ICD-10-CM codes for obstructed labor incorporate the reason for the obstruction into the code; therefore, only one code is required rather than two as in ICD-9-CM. For example, to code obstructed labor due to face presentation the following two ICD-9-CM codes are required: 660.0X, Obstruction caused by malposition of fetus at onset of labor and 652.4X, Face or brow presentation. In ICD-10-CM, only code O64.2XX-, Obstructed labor due to face presentation, is coded.

---

**Activity – Chapter 15 Organization and Classification**

In order to gain a better understanding of modifications to the organization, terminology, and classification of pregnancy, childbirth, and the puerperium conditions in ICD-10-CM, open the Tabular List. Review and compare the following entries and identify their differences.

| ICD-10-CM | ICD-9-CM |
|---|---|
| O12.1 | 646.2 |
| O15 | 642.6 |
| O80 | 650 |

---

# Chapter 16: Certain conditions originating in the perinatal period (P00-P96)

Chapter 16 of ICD-10-CM includes categories P00-P96 arranged in the following blocks:

| | |
|---|---|
| P00-P04 | Newborn affected by maternal factors and by complications of pregnancy, labor and delivery |
| P05-P08 | Disorders related to length of gestation and fetal growth |
| P09 | Abnormal findings on neonatal screening |
| P10-P15 | Birth trauma |
| P19-P29 | Respiratory and cardiovascular disorders specific to the perinatal period |
| P35-P39 | Infections specific to the perinatal period |
| P50-P61 | Hemorrhagic and hematological disorders of newborn |
| P70-P74 | Transitory endocrine and metabolic disorders specific to newborn |
| P76-P78 | Digestive system disorders of newborn |
| P80-P83 | Conditions involving the integument and temperature regulation of newborn |
| P84 | Other problems with newborn |
| P90-P96 | Other disorders originating in the perinatal period |

A number of new subchapters have been added to Chapter 16 for certain conditions originating in the perinatal period.

> **Note:** Codes for respiratory and cardiovascular disorders specific to the perinatal period are grouped together in block P19-P29.

Chapter 16 of ICD-10-CM also contains terminology updates. The first block in ICD-10-CM, newborns affected by maternal factors and by complications of pregnancy, labor, and delivery, the phrase "suspected to be" is included in the code title as a nonessential modifier to indicate that the codes are for use when the listed maternal condition is specified as the cause of confirmed or suspected newborn morbidity or potential morbidity.

> *Examples:*
> P00.3, Newborn (suspected to be) affected by other maternal circulatory and respiratory diseases
> P00.4, Newborn (suspected to be) affected by maternal nutritional disorders
> P00.5, Newborn (suspected to be) affected by maternal injury

Some revisions to the classification have occurred as well. For instance, the subclassification for 2,500 g and over for birth weight is no longer an option for category P05, Disorders of newborn related to slow growth and fetal malnutrition.

> **Activity – Chapter 16 Organization and Classification**
> In order to gain a better understanding of modifications to the organization, terminology, and classification of certain conditions originating in the perinatal period, reference the ICD-10-CM Tabular List, locate the following categories, and determine the revision.
>
> | ICD-10-CM | ICD-9-CM |
> |---|---|
> | P07.2 | 765.2 |
> | P36 | 771.81 |
> | P76.0 | 777.1 |

# Chapter 17: Congenital malformations, deformations and chromosomal abnormalities (Q00-Q99)

Chapter 17 of ICD-10-CM includes categories Q00-Q99 arranged in the following blocks:

Q00-Q07     Congenital malformations of the nervous system
Q10-Q18     Congenital malformations of eye, ear, face and neck
Q20-Q28     Congenital malformations of the circulatory system
Q30-Q34     Congenital malformations of the respiratory system
Q35-Q37     Cleft lip and cleft palate
Q38-Q45     Other congenital malformations of the digestive system
Q50-Q56     Congenital malformations of genital organs
Q60-Q64     Congenital malformations of the urinary system
Q65-Q79     Congenital malformations and deformations of the musculoskeletal system
Q80-Q89     Other congenital malformations
Q90-Q99     Chromosomal abnormalities, not elsewhere classified

The arrangement of ICD-10-CM's Chapter 17 is an improvement over ICD-9-CM's Chapter 14. Congenital malformations, deformations, and chromosomal abnormalities have been grouped into subchapters or blocks making it easier to identify the type of conditions classified to Chapter 17.

Modifications have also been made to specific categories that bring the terminology up-to-date with current medical practice.

---

*Example:*

**Q61     Cystic kidney disease**
Q61.0, Congenital renal cyst
Q61.1, Polycystic kidney, infantile type
Q61.2, Polycystic kidney, adult type

---

Other enhancements to Chapter 17 include classification changes that provide greater specificity than found in ICD-9-CM.

---

*Examples:*
Q35.1, Cleft hard palate
Q35.3, Cleft soft palate
Q35.5, Cleft hard palate with cleft soft palate
Q35.7, Cleft uvula
Q35.9, Cleft palate, unspecified

---

**Activity – Chapter 17 Organization and Classification**
To expand your knowledge of the alterations made to the organization, terminology, and classification of congenital malformations, deformations, and chromosomal abnormalities refer to the ICD-10-CM Tabular List, find the following codes or categories, and review the changes that were made between ICD revisions.

| ICD-10-CM | ICD-9-CM |
|---|---|
| Q53/Q55.22 | 752.5 |
| Q65-Q79 | 754 |
| Q90/Q91 | 758 |

# Chapter 18: Symptoms, signs and abnormal clinical and laboratory findings, not elsewhere classified (R00-R99)

Chapter 18 of ICD-10-CM includes categories R00-R99 arranged in the following blocks:

| | |
|---|---|
| R00-R09 | Symptoms and signs involving the circulatory and respiratory systems |
| R10-R19 | Symptoms and signs involving the digestive system and abdomen |
| R20-R23 | Symptoms and signs involving the skin and subcutaneous tissue |
| R25-R29 | Symptoms and signs involving the nervous and musculoskeletal systems |
| R30-R39 | Symptoms and signs involving the genitourinary system |
| R40-R46 | Symptoms and signs involving cognition, perception, emotional state and behavior |
| R47-R49 | Symptoms and signs involving speech and voice |
| R50-R69 | General symptoms and signs |
| R70-R79 | Abnormal findings on examination of blood, without diagnosis |
| R80-R82 | Abnormal findings on examination of urine, without diagnosis |
| R83-R89 | Abnormal findings on examination of other body fluids, substances and tissues, without diagnosis |
| R90-R94 | Abnormal findings on diagnostic imaging and in function studies, without diagnosis |
| R97 | Abnormal tumor markers |
| R99 | Ill-defined and unknown cause of mortality |

Chapter 18 of ICD-10-CM has undergone some organizational changes. For example, in ICD-10-CM codes for general symptoms and signs follow those related specifically to a body system or other relevant grouping.

In the comparison of Chapter 18 of ICD-10-CM to Chapter 16 of ICD-9-CM it is evident that some codes have been moved from one chapter to another.

---

*Examples:*

| | |
|---|---|
| ICD-9-CM (Chapter 7) | 427.89, Other specified cardiac dysrythmias |
| ICD-10-CM (Chapter 18) | R00.1, Bradycardia, unspecified |
| | |
| ICD-9-CM (Chapter 8) | 511.0, Pleurisy without mention of effusion or current tuberculosis |
| ICD-10-CM (Chapter 18) | R09.1, Pleurisy |
| | |
| ICD-9-CM (Chapter 9) | 527.7, Disturbance of salivary secretion |
| ICD-10-CM (Chapter 18) | R68.2, Dry mouth, unspecified |

---

A fairly substantial classification change was made to hematuria. Various types of hematuria are coded in Chapter 18 unless included with the underlying condition such as acute cystitis with hematuria. In those cases, the code is found in Chapter 14, Diseases of the genitourinary system.

**Activity – Chapter 18 Organization and Classification**
To increase your understanding of the revisions to the organization, terminology, and classification of symptoms, signs, and abnormal clinical and laboratory findings, refer to the ICD-10-CM Tabular List, review the listed categories or codes, and determine the modification by evaluating the ICD-9-CM information against what was found for the ICD-10-CM category or code.

| *ICD-10-CM* | *ICD-9-CM* |
|---|---|
| R10 | 789.0 |
| R41.81 | 797 |
| R90-R94 | 793/794 |

## *Chapter 19: Injury, poisoning and certain other consequences of external causes (S00-T88)*

As previously mentioned, a significant modification was made to the organization of Chapter 19. Type of injury is the first axis of classification for the injuries in ICD-9-CM whereas specific types of injuries found in categories S00-S99 of Chapter 19 are arranged by body region beginning with the head and concluding with the ankle and foot. This results in the grouping of injury types together under the site where it occurred.

| | |
|---|---|
| S00-S09 | Injuries to the head |
| S10-S19 | Injuries to the neck |
| S20-S29 | Injuries to the thorax |
| S30-S39 | Injuries to the abdomen, lower back, lumbar spine, pelvis and external genitals |
| S40-S49 | Injuries to the shoulder and upper arm |
| S50-S59 | Injuries to the elbow and forearm |
| S60-S69 | Injuries to the wrist, hand and fingers |
| S70-S79 | Injuries to the hip and thigh |
| S80-S89 | Injuries to the knee and lower leg |
| S90-S99 | Injuries to the ankle and foot |
| T07 | Injuries involving multiple body regions |
| T14 | Injury of unspecified body region |
| T15-T19 | Effects of foreign body entering through natural orifice |
| T20-T32 | Burns and corrosions |
| T20-T25 | Burns and corrosions of external body surface, specified by site |
| T26-T28 | Burns and corrosions confined to eye and internal organs |
| T30-T32 | Burns and corrosions of multiple and unspecified body regions |
| T33-T34 | Frostbite |
| T36-T50 | Poisoning by, adverse effect of and underdosing of drugs, medicaments and biological substances |
| T51-T65 | Toxic effects of substances chiefly nonmedicinal as to source |
| T66-T78 | Other and unspecified effects of external causes |
| T79 | Certain early complications of trauma |
| T80-T88 | Complications of surgical and medical care, not elsewhere classified |

In addition, generally the listings of conditions that follow the site are as follows:
- Superficial injury
- Open wound
- Fracture
- Dislocation and sprain
- Injury of nerves
- Injury of blood vessels
- Injury of muscle and tendon
- Crushing injury
- Traumatic amputation
- Other and unspecified injuries

Some categories in Chapter 19 have undergone title changes to reflect terminology in use today.

**Note:** ICD-10-CM uses the terms "displaced" and "nondisplaced" in the code descriptors while these terms were not used in ICD-9-CM.

In ICD-10-CM, codes from blocks T20-T32 classify burns and corrosions. The addition of the term "corrosion" is new in ICD-10-CM. The burn codes identify thermal burns, except for sunburns, that come from a heat source. The burn codes are also for burns resulting from electricity and radiation. Corrosions are burns due to chemicals.

A significant classification change was made to poisonings by and adverse effects of drugs, medicaments, and biological substances (T36-T50). ICD-10-CM does not provide different category codes to identify poisonings versus adverse effect. Instead under a single category for a specific drug are codes for poisonings, adverse effects, and underdosing of drugs, medicaments and biological substances. "Underdosing" is a new term in ICD-10-CM and is defined as taking less of a medication than is prescribed by a provider or the manufacturer's instructions with a resulting negative health consequence.

*Example:*
**T46.1  Poisoning by, adverse effect of, and underdosing of calcium-channel blockers**
T46.1X1, Poisoning by calcium-channel blocker, accidental (unintentional)
T46.1X2, Poisoning by calcium-channel blocker, intentional self-harm
T46.1X3, Poisoning by calcium-channel blocker, assault
T46.1X4, Poisoning by calcium-channel blocker, undetermined
T46.1X5, Adverse effect of calcium-channel blocker
T46.1X6, Underdosing of calcium-channel blocker

**Coding Tip:** Sequencing issues and problems are eliminated because poisonings, adverse effects, and underdosing are combination codes.

**Activity – Chapter 19 Organization and Classification**
For additional practice with learning the organizational, terminology, and classification changes to the chapter on injury, poisoning, and certain other consequences of external causes, refer to the ICD-10-CM Tabular List, refer to the below category or code, and ascertain the modification.

| ICD-10-CM | ICD-9-CM |
|-----------|----------|
| S12.0 | 805.01 |
| S41 | 880 |
| S43.50 | 840.0 |

## Chapter 20: External causes of morbidity (V00-Y99)

Chapter 20 of ICD-10-CM includes categories V00-Y99 arranged in the following blocks:

| | |
|---|---|
| V00-X58 | Accidents |
| V00-V99 | Transport accidents |
| V00-V09 | Pedestrian injured in transport accident |
| V10-V19 | Pedal cycle rider injured in transport accident |
| V20-V29 | Motorcycle rider injured in transport accident |
| V30-V39 | Occupant of three-wheeled motor vehicle injured in transport accident |
| V40-V49 | Car occupant injured in transport accident |
| V50-V59 | Occupant of pick-up truck or van injured in transport accident |
| V60-V69 | Occupant of heavy transport vehicle injured in transport accident |
| V70-V79 | Bus occupant injured in transport accident |
| V80-V89 | Other land transport accidents |
| V90-V94 | Water transport accidents |
| V95-V97 | Air and space transport accidents |
| V98-V99 | Other and unspecified transport accidents |
| W00-X58 | Other external causes of accidental injury |
| W00-W19 | Slipping, tripping, stumbling and falls |
| W20-W49 | Exposure to inanimate mechanical forces |
| W50-W64 | Exposure to animate mechanical forces |
| W65-W74 | Accidental non-transport drowning and submersion |
| W85-W99 | Exposure to electric current, radiation and extreme ambient air temperature and pressure |
| X00-X08 | Exposure to smoke, fire and flames |
| X10-X19 | Contact with heat and hot substances |
| X30-X39 | Exposure to forces of nature |
| X52-X58 | Accidental exposure to other specified factors |
| X71-X83 | Intentional self-harm |
| X92-Y08 | Assault |
| Y21-Y33 | Event of undetermined intent |
| Y35-Y38 | Legal intervention, operations of war, military operations and terrorism |
| Y62-Y84 | Complications of medical and surgical care |
| Y62-Y69 | Misadventures to patients during surgical and medical care |
| Y70-Y82 | Medical devices associated with adverse incidents in diagnostic and therapeutic use |
| Y83-Y84 | Surgical and other medical procedures as the cause of abnormal reaction of the patient, or of later complication, without mention of misadventure at the time of the procedure |
| Y90-Y99 | Supplementary factors related to causes of morbidity classified elsewhere |

As previously noted, codes for external causes are no longer found in a supplemental classification in ICD-10-CM. The causes currently located in the ICD-9-CM E code chapter have been disseminated to Chapter 19: Injury, poisoning and certain other consequences of external causes, or Chapter 20: External causes of morbidity. Codes in Chapter 20 capture the cause of the injury or health condition, the intent (unintentional or accidental; or intentional, such as suicide or assault), the place where the event occurred, the activity of the patient at the time of the event, and the person's status (namely civilian, military).

Changes in terminology were also necessary due to the revisions made overall to this chapter.

---

**Note:** ICD-10-CM category V45 is titled "Car occupant injured in collision with railway train or railway vehicle" while the title of ICD-9-CM category E810 is "Motor vehicle traffic accident involving collision with train."

---

In numerous instances, conditions included as subcategory codes in ICD-9-CM have been given a specific category code in ICD-10-CM allowing expansion of the codes at the fourth-, fifth-, or sixth-character level.

---

*Example:*
ICD-9-CM      E884.0, Fall from playground equipment
ICD-10-CM    W09,    Fall on and from playground equipment
                      W09.0, Fall on or from playground slide
                      W09.1, Fall from playground swing
                      W09.2, Fall on or from jungle gym
                      W09.8, Fall on or from other playground equipment

---

**Activity – Chapter 20 Organization and Classification**
To find out more about the organization, terminology, and classification modifications to external causes of morbidity, refer to the ICD-10-CM Tabular List, locate the listed ICD-10-CM category or code, evaluate the ICD-9-CM information against what was found, and discern the variances.

| *ICD-10-CM* | *ICD-9-CM* |
|---|---|
| W00-W19 | E880-E888 |
| W54-W64 | E905-E906 |
| Y38 | E979 |

# Chapter 21: Factors influencing health status and contact with health services (Z00-Z99)

Coding professionals will find the listing of codes for factors influencing health status and contact with health services a bit different in ICD-10-CM than what is currently found in ICD-9-CM. The following blocks represent the ICD-10-CM arrangement:

| | |
|---|---|
| Z00-Z13 | Persons encountering health services for examinations |
| Z14-Z15 | Genetic carrier and genetic susceptibility to disease |
| Z16 | Resistance to antimicrobial drugs |
| Z17 | Estrogen receptor status |
| Z18 | Retained foreign body fragment |
| Z20-Z28 | Persons with potential health hazards related to communicable diseases |
| Z30-Z39 | Persons encountering health services in circumstances related to reproduction |
| Z40-Z53 | Encounters for other specific health care |
| Z55-Z65 | Persons with potential health hazards related to socioeconomic and psychosocial circumstances |
| Z66 | Do not resuscitate status |
| Z67 | Blood type |
| Z68 | Body mass index (BMI) |
| Z69-Z76 | Persons encountering health services in other circumstances |
| Z77-Z99 | Persons with potential health hazards related to family and personal history and certain conditions influencing health status |

Some categories in Chapter 21 have rephrased titles to better reflect the situations the codes classify.

---

**Note:** The description for Z08 is "Encounter for follow-up examination after completed treatment for malignant neoplasm" compared to ICD-9-CM code title for V67.2 "Follow-up examination following chemotherapy."

---

An example of decreased specificity in ICD-10-CM is code Z23, Encounter for immunization. This code is not further classified. In ICD-9-CM, category codes V03, V04, V05, and V06 are used to identify the types of immunizations.

---

**Activity – Chapter 21 Organization and Classification**

To become more familiar with other revisions to the organization, terminology, and classifications of factors influencing health status and contact with health services, refer to the ICD-10-CM Tabular list, find the ICD-10-CM category or code for those listed here, and assess how it differs from ICD-9-CM.

| ICD-10-CM | ICD-9-CM |
|---|---|
| Z33.2 | 635 |
| Z91.010 | V15.01 |
| Z96 | V43 |

## Section 8 – Chapter 15–21 Guidelines

This section is designed to highlight the revisions to the guidelines found in Chapters 15–21 of ICD-10-CM. All modifications have not been illustrated but certain guiding principles have been selected to show guideline variations from ICD-9-CM. Also included in this section is the review of chapter-specific coding guidelines published by NCHS.

## *Chapter 15: Pregnancy, childbirth and the puerperium (O00-O9A)*

At the beginning of Chapter 15 are guidelines that provide instructions for coding professionals.

> **Note:** Codes from this chapter are for use only on maternal records, never on newborn records.

> **Note:** Trimesters are counted from the first day of the last menstrual period. They are defined as follows:
> - 1st trimester – less than 14 weeks 0 days
> - 2nd trimester – 14 weeks 0 days to less than 28 weeks 0 days
> - 3rd trimester – 28 weeks 0 days until delivery

These guidelines should be followed when selecting a code from this chapter.

There are guideline changes to a number of codes in this chapter as well.

| | |
|---|---|
| *Examples:* | |
| ICD-9-CM | For category 643, Excessive vomiting in pregnancy, early vomiting and late vomiting are differentiated by 22 completed weeks |
| ICD-10-CM | For category O21, Excessive vomiting in pregnancy, early vomiting and late vomiting are differentiated by 20 completed weeks |
| ICD-9-CM | For category 640, hemorrhage in early pregnancy is defined as hemorrhage before completion of 22 weeks gestation |
| ICD-10-CM | For category O20, hemorrhage in early pregnancy is defined as hemorrhage before completion of 20 weeks of gestation |

The NCHS has published chapter-specific guidelines for Chapter 15 of ICD-10-CM:
- Guideline I.C.15.a. General rules for obstetric cases
- Guideline I.C.15.b. Selection of OB principal or first-listed diagnosis
- Guideline I.C.15.c. Pre-existing conditions versus conditions due to the pregnancy
- Guideline I.C.15.d. Pre-existing hypertension in pregnancy
- Guideline I.C.15.e. Fetal conditions affecting the management of the mother
- Guideline I.C.15.f. HIV infection in pregnancy, childbirth and the puerperium
- Guideline I.C.15.g. Diabetes mellitus in pregnancy
- Guideline I.C.15.h. Long-term use of insulin
- Guideline I.C.15.i. Gestational (pregnancy induced) diabetes
- Guideline I.C.15.j. Sepsis and septic shock complicating abortion, pregnancy, childbirth and the puerperium
- Guideline I.C.15.k. Puerperal sepsis
- Guideline I.C.15.l. Alcohol and tobacco use during pregnancy, childbirth and the puerperium

- Guideline I.C.15.m. Poisoning, toxic effects, adverse effects and underdosing in a pregnant patient
- Guideline I.C.15.n. Normal delivery, code O80
- Guideline I.C.15.o. The peripartum and postpartum periods
- Guideline I.C.15.p. Code O94, sequelae of complications of pregnancy, childbirth and the puerperium
- Guideline I.C.15.q. Abortions
- Guideline I.C.15.r. Abuse in pregnant patient

---

**Activity – Chapter 15 Guidelines**

To gain an understanding of these rules, access the 2013 guidelines from the NCHS website (http://www.cdc.gov/nchs/icd/icd10cm.htm) and read Chapter 15: Pregnancy, childbirth and the puerperium guidelines I.C.15.a.1 through I.C.15.r on pages 51–59.

---

## *Chapter 16: Certain conditions originating in the perinatal period (P00-P96)*

Throughout Chapter 16 are new notes that help to clarify how codes are to be used.

---

*Examples:*

The following note appears under P07: When both birth weight and gestational age of the newborn are available, both should be coded with birth weight sequenced before gestational age.

The following note appears under P08.21: Newborn with gestation period over 40 completed weeks to 42 completed weeks.

---

Codes from this chapter are only for use on the newborn or infant record, never on the maternal record as indicated by a note that appears at the beginning of Chapter 16. Codes from this chapter are also only applicable for liveborn infants. Further, should a condition originate in the perinatal period and continue throughout the life of the child, the perinatal code should continue to be used regardless of the age of the patient as explained by an introductory note to Chapter 16.

The NCHS has published chapter-specific guidelines for Chapter 16 of ICD-10-CM:
- Guideline I.C.16.a. General perinatal rules
- Guideline I.C.16.b. Observation and evaluation of newborns for suspected conditions not found
- Guideline I.C.16.c. Coding additional perinatal diagnoses
- Guideline I.C.16.d. Prematurity and fetal growth retardation
- Guideline I.C.16.e. Low birth weight and immaturity status
- Guideline I.C.16.f. Bacterial sepsis of newborn
- Guideline I.C.16.g. Stillbirth

---

**Activity – Chapter 16 Guidelines**

To gain an understanding of these rules, access the 2013 guidelines from the NCHS website (http://www.cdc.gov/nchs/icd/icd10cm.htm) and read Chapter 16: Newborn (perinatal) guidelines I.C.16.a through I.C.16.g on pages 60–62.

---

## *Chapter 17: Congenital malformations, deformations and chromosomal abnormalities (Q00-Q99)*

Additional guideline modifications were made to specific codes. For example, in ICD-9-CM certain congenital malformations of the anterior segment of the eye do not have any instructions for code usage listed below codes 743.44 or 743.45. In contrast, guidelines for code Q13.1 and Q13.81 state to use an additional code for associated glaucoma.

Congenital anomalies or syndromes may occur as a set of symptoms or multiple malformations. If there is no specific code, a code should be assigned for each manifestation of the syndrome, from any chapter in the classification. For syndromes with specific codes, additional codes may be assigned to identify manifestations not included in the specific code.

The NCHS has published chapter-specific guidelines for Chapter 17 of ICD-10-CM:
- Guideline I.C.17. Congenital malformations, deformations and chromosomal abnormalities (Q00-Q99)

**Activity – Chapter 17 Guidelines**
To gain an understanding of these rules, access the 2013 guidelines from the NCHS website (http://www.cdc.gov/nchs/icd/icd10cm.htm) and read Chapter 17: Congenital malformations, deformations and chromosomal abnormalities guideline I.C.17 on pages 62–63.

## *Chapter 18: Symptoms, signs and abnormal clinical and laboratory findings, not elsewhere classified (R00-R99)*

A lengthy guideline appears at the beginning of Chapter 18 in ICD-10-CM outlining the conditions classified to this chapter. Additionally, guidelines for code usage appear at the subchapter level.

---

**Note:** Many of the new blocks and categories in chapter 18 have extensive *Excludes1* notes such as the one found under R09, Other symptoms and signs involving the circulatory and respiratory system.

---

New guidelines that clarify code usage are also found under specific codes. Code R52, Pain unspecified, includes inclusive terms and *Excludes1* notes.

The NCHS has published chapter-specific guidelines for Chapter 18 of ICD-10-CM:
- Guideline I.C.18.a. Use of symptom codes
- Guideline I.C.18.b. Use of a symptom code with a definitive diagnosis code
- Guideline I.C.18.c. Combination codes that include symptoms
- Guideline I.C.18.d. Repeated falls
- Guideline I.C.18.e. Coma scale
- Guideline I.C.18.f. Functional quadriplegia
- Guideline I.C.18.g. SIRS due to non-infectious process
- Guideline I.C.18.h. Death NOS

---

**Activity – Chapter 18 Guidelines**

To gain an understanding of these rules, access the 2013 guidelines from the NCHS website (http://www.cdc.gov/nchs/icd/icd10cm.htm) and read Chapter 18: Symptoms, signs and abnormal clinical and laboratory findings, not elsewhere classified guidelines I.C.18.a through I.C.18.h on pages 63–65.

---

# Chapter 19: Injury, poisoning and certain other consequences of external causes (S00-T88)

The following guideline appears at the beginning of Chapter 19: Use secondary code(s) from Chapter 20, External causes of morbidity, to indicate cause of injury. Codes within the T section that include the external cause do not require an additional external cause code.

Instructions for coding open wounds have changed in ICD-10-CM. The note in ICD-9-CM defines "complicated" used in the fourth-digit subdivisions to mean those open wounds with infection. ICD-10-CM contains a note under the different categories for open wounds and directs the coding professional to code also any associated wound infection.

A similar change has occurred to the instruction for complications of surgical and medical care, not elsewhere classified (T80-T88). In ICD-9-CM, there is no guideline under this subchapter. However, ICD-10-CM includes a note stating to use an additional code (Y62-Y82) to identify devices involved and details of circumstances.

---

**Note:** Most categories in Chapter 19 have seventh characters that identify the encounter:
A      initial encounter
D      subsequent encounter
S      sequela

---

Additional seventh characters are available to identify specific encounters for fracture coding. Seventh characters for fractures are unique to each type of bone and type of fracture.

---

**Coding Tip:** It is necessary to review the fracture seventh characters carefully before assigning a seventh character.

---

The NCHS has published chapter-specific guidelines for Chapter 19 of ICD-10-CM:
- Guideline I.C.19.a. Seventh characters
- Guideline I.C.19.b. Coding of injuries
- Guideline I.C.19.c. Coding of traumatic fractures
- Guideline I.C.19.d. Coding of burns and corrosions
- Guideline I.C.19.e. Adverse effects, poisoning, underdosing and toxic effects
- Guideline I.C.19.f. Adult and child abuse, neglect and other maltreatment
- Guideline I.C.19.g. Complications of care

---

**Activity – Chapter 19 Guidelines**
To gain an understanding of these rules, access the 2013 guidelines from the NCHS website (http://www.cdc.gov/nchs/icd/icd10cm.htm) and read Chapter 19: Injury, poisoning and certain other consequences of external causes guidelines I.C.19.a through I.C.19.g.5 on pages 65–74.

---

## *Chapter 20: External causes of morbidity (V00-Y99)*

New notes have been added in Chapter 20 to indicate which categories require the seventh character to indicate whether the episode of care being identified was the initial, subsequent, or a secondary consequence or result (sequelae).

While there is an instructional note found at the start of category E849, place of occurrence, in ICD-9-CM, it has been expanded in ICD-10-CM. The new guidelines state to use Y92 in conjunction with the activity code and the place of occurrence should be recorded only at the initial encounter for treatment.

> **Coding Tip:** Use an activity code from category Y93 in addition to the place of occurrence code from category Y92.

The NCHS has published chapter-specific guidelines for Chapter 20 of ICD-10-CM:
- Guideline I.C.20.a. General external cause coding guidelines
- Guideline I.C.20.b. Place of occurrence guideline
- Guideline I.C.20.c. Activity code
- Guideline I.C.20.d. Place of occurrence, activity, and status codes used with other external cause code
- Guideline I.C.20.e. If the reporting format limits the number of external cause codes
- Guideline I.C.20.f. Multiple external cause coding guidelines
- Guideline I.C.20.g. Child and adult abuse guideline
- Guideline I.C.20.h. Unknown or undetermined intent guideline
- Guideline I.C.20.i. Sequela (late effects) of external cause guidelines
- Guideline I.C.20.j. Terrorism guidelines
- Guideline I.C.20.k. External cause status

**Activity – Chapter 20 Guidelines**
To gain an understanding of these rules, access the 2013 guidelines from the NCHS website (http://www.cdc.gov/nchs/icd/icd10cm.htm) and read Chapter 20: External causes of morbidity guidelines I.C.20.a through I.C.20.k on pages 75–80.

# Chapter 21: Factors influencing health status and contact with health services (Z00-Z99)

The note at the beginning of this chapter has been modified from what it states in ICD-9-CM. All codes in Chapter 21 are affected by these revised guidelines. Here is the note:

> Z codes represent reasons for encounters. A corresponding procedure code must accompany a Z code if a procedure is performed. Categories Z00-Z99 are provided for occasions when circumstances other than a disease, injury or external cause classifiable to categories A00-Y89 are recorded as 'diagnoses' or 'problems'. This can arise in two main ways:
>
> a) When a person who may or may not be sick encounters the health services for some specific purpose, such as to receive limited care or service for a current condition, to donate an organ or tissue, to receive prophylactic vaccination (immunization), or to discuss a problem which is in itself not a disease or injury.
>
> b) When some circumstance or problem is present which influences the person's health status but is not in itself a current illness or injury.

Instructional notes also have been added to different categories to explain how codes should be assigned.

---

*Examples:*

Under category Z01, Encounter for other special examination without complaint, suspected or reported diagnosis, is the following note: Codes from category Z01 represent the reason for the encounter. A separate procedure code is required to identify any examination or procedure performed.

Under category Z85, Personal history of malignant neoplasm, is the following note: Code first any follow-up examination after treatment of malignant neoplasm (Z08).

---

The NCHS has published chapter-specific guidelines for Chapter 21 of ICD-10-CM:
- Guideline I.C.21.a. Use of Z codes in any healthcare setting
- Guideline I.C.21.b. Z codes indicate a reason for an encounter
- Guideline I.C.21.c. Categories of Z codes

---

**Activity – Chapter 21 Guidelines**

To gain an understanding of these rules, access the 2013 guidelines from the NCHS website (http://www.cdc.gov/nchs/icd/icd10cm.htm) and read Chapter 21: Factors influencing health status and contact with health services guidelines I.C.21.a through I.C.21.c on pages 80–95.

# Sections 7 and 8 Review Questions

1. True or false? An injury code with the seventh character D for subsequent encounter may be used for as long as a patient is receiving treatment for an injury.
   a. True
   b. False

2. True or false? If a patient has both an open wound of the shoulder and an associated wound infection, only one code is assigned in both ICD-9-CM and ICD-10-CM.
   a. True
   b. False

3. ICD-10-CM contains codes for all but one of the following conditions:
   a. Eclampsia in labor
   b. Eclampsia in the puerperium
   c. Eclampsia in the first trimester
   d. Eclampsia in the second trimester

4. What is the correct ICD-10-CM code(s) for severe generalized abdominal pain with abdominal rigidity?
   a. R19.3
   b. R10.0
   c. R10.84
   d. R19.3, R10.0

5. What is the purpose of the fifth character for category Y38, Terrorism?
   a. A placeholder
   b. To identify the person injured
   c. As a way to indicate place of occurrence
   d. To classify the encounter

6. True or false? Before assigning codes from the ICD-10-CM chapter on pregnancy, childbirth and the puerperium, coding professionals need to determine if a condition was pre-existing prior to pregnancy or developed during the pregnancy in order to select the correct code.
   a. True
   b. False

7. Codes for bacterial sepsis of newborn are found in which block in Chapter 16?
   a. P90-P96, Other disorders originating in the perinatal period
   b. P50-P61, Hemorrhagic and hematological disorders of newborn
   c. P84, Other problems with newborn
   d. P35-P39, Infections specific to the perinatal period

8. True or false? Codes from the ICD-10-CM chapter on congenital malformations, deformations and chromosomal abnormalities may be used only up until the 28th day following birth.
   a. True
   b. False

9. If a condition is discovered during a screening, the screening code is:
   a. Not assigned
   b. Assigned but coded secondary to the condition discovered
   c. Assigned with the condition discovered coded secondary
   d. Assigned without a code for the discovered condition

10. True or false? ICD-10-CM placed a single category of codes for poisonings, adverse effects of and underdosing of drugs, medicaments, and biological substances.
    a. True
    b. False

# Final Review Questions

1.  The final rule to adopt ICD-10-CM and ICD-10-PCS states the compliance date for ICD-10-CM is:
    a.  October 1, 2013
    b.  January 16, 2009
    c.  October 1, 2014
    d.  January 1, 2014

2.  All of the following are new features of ICD-10-CM, *except:*
    a.  Injuries are grouped by body part rather than by categories of injuries
    b.  The concept of laterality has been added
    c.  Newly recognized conditions and conditions that are not uniquely identified in ICD-9-CM have been given codes
    d.  Codes for intraoperative complications and postprocedural disorders have been combined

3.  According to the note under Chapter 18: Symptoms, signs and abnormal clinical and laboratory findings, not elsewhere classified, categories in this chapter include signs and symptoms that point rather definitely to a given diagnosis.
    a.  True
    b.  False

4.  ICD-10-CM and ICD-9-CM have similar structures in which of the following?
    a.  Hypertension table
    b.  Note placement
    c.  Morphology appendix
    d.  All of the above

5.  What is the purpose of the X placeholder in category X78?
    a.  To code to the highest level of specificity
    b.  As a placeholder for future expansion
    c.  As filler so a seventh character may be assigned
    d.  To provide further specificity about the condition being coded

6.  ICD-10-CM code N30.01, Acute cystitis with hematuria, represents which use of a combination code?
    a.  Two diagnoses
    b.  A diagnosis with an associated sign or symptom
    c.  A diagnosis with an associated complication
    d.  All of the above

7.  Codes in Chapter 20, External causes of morbidity, identify all of the following *except:*
    a.  Intent (unintentional/accidental, intentional self-harm or assault)
    b.  Place where the event occurred
    c.  Activity of the patient at the time of the event
    d.  Poisoning by medicaments and biological substances

8.  A patient with a diagnosis of interstitial cystitis due to E coli with hematuria is coded:
    a.  N30.11, N02.9
    b.  N30.10, N02.9, B96.20
    c.  N30.11, B96.20
    d.  N30.91, B96.20

9.  ICD-10-CM category J44 is used to classify all but the following:
    a.  Chronic asthmatic (obstructive) bronchitis
    b.  Asthmatic bronchitis
    c.  Chronic obstructive asthma
    d.  Chronic obstructive pulmonary disease

10. What is the correct ICD-10-CM code for acute nonsuppurative otitis media, right ear?
    a.  H65.91
    b.  H65.111
    c.  H65.199
    d.  H65.191

11. A patient with a diagnosis of fatigue fracture of vertebra, lumbar region, and subsequent encounter for fracture with delayed healing is coded:
    a.  M48.46G
    b.  M48.46XG
    c.  M48.45XG
    d.  M48.47XG

12. True or false? Uncontrolled hypertension and controlled hypertension have different codes in ICD-10-CM.
    a.  True
    b.  False

13. According to NCHS Guidelines, which of the following is the default for a patient with a diagnosis of right-side hemiplegia, ICD-10-CM category G81?
    a.  Dominant side
    b.  Nondominant side
    c.  Unspecified side
    d.  Right side

14. ICD-10-CM code H40.0 is used to classify:
    a.  Glaucoma suspect
    b.  Ocular hypertension
    c.  Borderline glaucoma
    d.  All of the above

15. ICD-10-CM category Q35 does not contain a specific code for which of the following conditions in which ICD-9-CM does?
    a.  Bilateral cleft palate
    b.  Cleft soft palate
    c.  Cleft uvula
    d.  Cleft hard palate

16. True or false? Codes from categories P00-P04 may be assigned if testing or treatment is done and no problem with the infant is determined.
    a.  True
    b.  False

17. What documentation is necessary in order to choose the correct fifth character for post-traumatic urethral stricture?
    a.  Gender
    b.  Severity
    c.  Cause
    d.  Manifestation

18. For ICD-10-CM categories V00-V99, the type of vehicle the victim is an occupant in is identified in the:
    a. First two characters
    b. Last two characters
    c. Seventh character
    d. The placeholder X

19. True or false? If the abnormal test finding corresponds to a confirmed diagnosis, the abnormal test findings code should not be coded in addition to the confirmed diagnosis.
    a. True
    b. False

20. Codes from which category/categories is/are assigned for a patient who has suffered from an AMI and has a new AMI within the four-week time frame of the initial AMI?
    a. I21
    b. I22
    c. I21, I22
    d. I21, I25

# Part I: ICD-10-CM Diagnostic Coding

## *ICD-10-CM Resources – References*

2012 ICD-10-CM is available at http://www.cdc.gov/nchs/icd/icd10cm.htm or http://www.cms.hhs.gov/ICD10

- 2013 ICD-10-CM Index to Diseases and Injuries
- 2013 ICD-10-CM Tabular List of Diseases and Injuries
    - Instructional Notations
- 2013 Official Guidelines for Coding and Reporting
- 2013 Table of Drugs and Chemicals
- 2013 Neoplasm Table
- 2013 Index to External Causes
- 2013 Mapping "ICD-9-CM to ICD-10-CM" and "ICD-10-CM to ICD-9-CM"

*ICD-10-CM: The Complete Official Draft Code Set 2013* (Optum)
- Introduction
- ICD-10-CM Draft Conventions
- ICD-10-CM Draft Official Guidelines for Coding and Reporting (2013)
- ICD-10-CM Index to Diseases and Injuries
- ICD-10-CM Neoplasm Table
- ICD-10-CM Table of Drugs and Chemicals
- ICD-10-CM Index to External Causes
- ICD-10-CM Tabular List of Diseases and Injuries

# ICD-10-CM Coding Conventions and Coding Guidelines Review

## ICD-10-CM Coding Conventions

1.  The ICD-10-CM code for electrocution is T75.4 and requires the use of a seventh character to identify the encounter. Which of the following is the correct code for an initial encounter to treat the electrocution?
    a.    T75.4A
    b.    T75.4XA
    c.    T75.4XXA
    d.    T75.4

2.  Nonessential modifiers are enclosed in:
    a.    Boxes
    b.    Brackets
    c.    Parentheses
    d.    Colons

3.  True or false? When an *Excludes2* note appears under a code, it is acceptable to use both the code and the excluded code together.
    a.    True
    b.    False

4.  The first character of an ICD-10-CM code is:
    a.    Always a number
    b.    Always a letter
    c.    Can be either a number or letter
    d.    None of the above

5.  A(n) _____ note means "not coded here."
    a.    *Includes*
    b.    *Excludes2*
    c.    *Excludes1*
    d.    None of the above

6.  Codes titled "other" or "other specified" are to be used:
    a.    When the record itself is not available for review
    b.    When the information in the medical record provides detail for which a specific code does not exist
    c.    When only outpatient diagnostic records are being coded
    d.    When the information in the medical record is insufficient to assign a more specific code

7.  True or false? Similar to ICD-9-CM, in ICD-10-CM all categories are three characters.
    a.    True
    b.    False

8.  True or false? When the term "and" is used in a narrative statement it is interpreted to mean only "and."
    a.    True
    b.    False

9. True or false? In ICD-10-CM all inclusion notes contain all conditions for which a particular code number is to be used and are considered to be "exhaustive."
   a. True
   b. False

10. True or false? In ICD-10-CM a "code also" note provides sequencing guidance to the coding professional.
    a. True
    b. False

## ICD-10-CM Coding Guidelines

11. If an encounter is solely for chemotherapy, immunotherapy, or radiation therapy for a neoplastic condition, the first reported diagnosis is:
    a. The diagnosis toward which the treatment is directed
    b. The appropriate Z51 code
    c. Either a or b
    d. The diagnosis that the physician lists first on the order

12. True or false? When assigning the principal diagnosis for a patient with AIDS, the AIDS code would always be sequenced before any other conditions.
    a. True
    b. False

13. A patient has liver metastasis due to adenocarcinoma of the rectum which was resected two years ago. The patient has been receiving radiotherapy to the liver with some relief of pain. The patient is being admitted at this time for management of severe anemia due to the malignancy. The principal diagnosis listed on this admission is:
    a. Liver metastasis
    b. Adenocarcinoma of the rectum
    c. Anemia
    d. Admission for radiotherapy

14. True or false? Code P95, Stillbirth, is only for use for institutions that maintain separate records for stillborns and should never be used on the mother's record.
    a. True
    b. False

15. True or false? A fracture not described as "displaced" or "not displaced" by default should be coded as "not displaced."
    a. True
    b. False

16. A patient is admitted six weeks post-acute anterolateral myocardial infarction with a subsequent posterior acute MI. Which is the appropriate coding and sequencing for the encounter for the posterior acute MI in ICD-10-CM?
    a. I21.09, STEMI involving other coronary artery of anterior wall,
       I22.8, Subsequent STEMI of other sites
    b. I21.29, STEMI of other sites,
       I25.2, Old myocardial infarction
    c. I22.8, Subsequent STEMI of other sites;
       I21.09, STEMI involving other coronary artery of anterior wall
    d. I22.8, Subsequent STEMI of other sites,
       I25.2, Old myocardial infarction

17. When multiple burns are present, the first sequenced diagnosis is the:
    a. Burn that is treated surgically
    b. Burn that is closest to the head
    c. Highest-degree burn
    d. Any of the above

18. True or false? A place of occurrence code should be used only at the initial encounter for treatment.
    a. True
    b. False

19. In ICD-10-CM diabetes mellitus codes include:
    a. The type of diabetes mellitus
    b. The body system affected
    c. The complication affecting that body system
    d. All of the above

20. True or false? A causal relationship can be assumed in a patient with both coronary atherosclerosis and angina pectoris and thus, the appropriate combination code should be assigned.
    a. True
    b. False

21. True or false? Patients with a prior diagnosis of an HIV-related illness should be assigned the code for AIDS (B20) on every subsequent admission.
    a. True
    b. False

22. Which of the following would be assigned to code I11.0, Hypertensive heart disease with heart failure?
    a. Left heart failure with benign hypertension
    b. Hypertensive cardiomegaly
    c. Congestive heart failure due to hypertension
    d. All of the above would be assigned to code I11.0

23. When an OB patient enters the hospital for complications of pregnancy during one trimester and remains in the hospital into a subsequent trimester, the final character selected for the antepartum conditions should be:
    a. For the trimester in which the complication developed
    b. For the trimester in which the patient delivered
    c. For the trimester in which the patient was discharged
    d. Any trimester as long as the same character is used for all complications

24. True or false? In the case where a 20-day-old baby has a condition that may be either due to the birth process or community-acquired and there is no documentation to support either one, the default should be community-acquired rather than birth process.
    a. True
    b. False

25. True or false? Regardless of the number of external cause codes assigned on a particular record, there should be only one place of occurrence code and one activity code assigned to a record.
    a. True
    b. False

26. True or false? A noncompliance code or complication of care code is to be used with an underdosing code to indicate intent.
    a. True
    b. False

27. When reporting an encounter for a patient who is HIV positive but has never had any symptoms, the following code is assigned:
    a. B20, Human immunodeficiency virus [HIV] disease
    b. Z21, Asymptomatic HIV infection status
    c. R75, Inconclusive laboratory evidence of human immunodeficiency virus (HIV)
    d. Z20.6, Contact with and (suspected) exposure to HIV

28. In reviewing the medical record of a patient admitted for a left herniorrhaphy, the coder notes an extremely low potassium level on the laboratory report. In examining the physician's order, the coder notices that intravenous potassium was ordered. The physician has not listed any indication of an abnormal potassium level or any related condition within the medical record. The best course of action for the coder to take is to:
    a. Confer with the physician and ask if the condition should be listed as a final diagnosis
    b. Code the record as is
    c. Code the condition as an abnormal blood chemistry
    d. Code the abnormal potassium level as a complication following surgery

29. True or false? When coding severe sepsis a minimum of three codes is required.
    a. True
    b. False

30. When a patient seeks medical attention for an injury that occurred several days prior to the medical encounter, which is the appropriate seventh character?
    a. A, initial encounter
    b. D, subsequent encounter
    c. S, sequela
    d. No seventh character is used when there is delayed treatment

# Coding in ICD-10-CM

ICD-10-CM differs from ICD-9-CM in its organization and structure, code composition, and level of detail; however, many components stay the same. ICD-10-CM has the same hierarchical structure as ICD-9-CM, and all codes with the same first three characters have common traits. Each character beyond the first three adds more specificity. Even though ICD-10-CM has more characters (up to seven) and uses alpha characters, each code must be at least three characters, with a decimal point used after the third character. Most, but not all, three-character categories have been subdivided. Up to four characters may follow the decimal. However, not every code will have four characters after the decimal; the concept is the same as ICD-9-CM.

The first character of the ICD-10-CM code is an alpha character, and each letter is associated with a particular chapter, except for the letters **D** and **H**. The letter D is used in both Chapter 2: Neoplasms, and Chapter 3: Diseases of the blood and blood-forming organs and certain disorders involving the immune mechanism. The letter H is used in both Chapter 7: Diseases of the eye and adnexa, and Chapter 8: Diseases of the ear and mastoid process. To allow for future revisions or expansions of the classification, every available code is not used.

The letters I and O are used in ICD-10-CM, but they shouldn't be confused with the numbers 1 and 0 because the letters I and O are only used in the first character position and this character is always a letter.

| ICD-9-CM | ICD-10-CM |
|---|---|
| • Consists of three to five characters <br> • First digit is numeric but occasionally can be alpha (E or V) <br> • Second, third, fourth, and fifth digits are numeric <br> • Always at least three digits <br> • Decimal placed after the first three characters (or with E codes, placed after the first four characters) <br> • Alpha characters are not case-sensitive | • Consists of three to seven characters <br> • First character is always alpha <br> • All letters used except U <br> • Character 2 always numeric <br> • Characters 3 through 7 can be alpha or numeric <br> • Always at least three digits <br> • Decimal placed after the first three characters <br> • Alpha characters are not case-sensitive |

A few important changes to ICD-10-CM are listed here:
- ICD-10-CM consists of 21 chapters.
- The order of some chapters has been rearranged, with reclassification of some conditions.
- The addition of a sixth character in some chapters.
- A seventh character added in some chapters (primarily pregnancy, injury, and external cause chapters).
- ICD-10-CM includes full code titles for all codes (no references back to common fourth and fifth digits).
- No supplementary classifications, with all codes incorporated into main classification.
- Expansion of postoperative complications and a distinction made between intraoperative complications and postprocedural disorders.

- Category restructuring and code reorganization.
- A placeholder X is used in some codes to allow for future expansion and also to fill out empty characters when a code contains fewer than six characters and a seventh character applies.
- Instructional note, guideline, and time frame changes.
- Combination codes for conditions and common symptoms or manifestations have been added.
- Laterality (meaning left or right side) has been added where applicable.
- Seventh characters added for type of encounter (initial, subsequent, and sequela) for injuries and external causes.

## Coding and Use of Seventh Characters

While more detailed information will be provided later in this training, certain basic information is provided here so that correct seventh characters can be assigned throughout this training course when encountered.

Seventh characters have been added in some chapters, primarily in the obstetrics, injury, and external cause chapters. They may be either alpha or numeric and are added to the end of the code in the seventh position when applicable. They provide additional information about the characteristics of the encounter. Seventh characters have different meanings depending on the section, and the applicable values are available in the Tabular section of ICD-10-CM. The category will identify the necessity to use the seventh character. The applicable seventh character is required for all codes within that category, or as the notes in the Tabular List instruct. A code that has an applicable seventh character is considered invalid without the seventh character. The seventh character must always be the seventh character in the data field, and if the code is not six characters, a placeholder of X is required to fill empty characters.

The meanings of the seventh character vary across chapters and categories. In the Injury and External Cause chapters the seventh character identifies the encounter (initial, subsequent, sequela). Fracture codes include additional information that can be provided by the seventh character. See the Tabular List for the exact seventh characters available for fracture coding.

The seventh characters for "initial encounter" are used while the patient is receiving active treatment of the condition. Examples of active treatment are: surgical treatment, emergency department encounter, and evaluation and treatment by a new physician.

The seventh characters for "subsequent encounter" are used for encounters after the patient has received active treatment of the condition and is receiving routine care for the condition during the healing or recovery phase. Examples of subsequent care are: cast change or removal, removal of external or internal fixation device, medication adjustment, other aftercare and follow-up visits following treatment of the injury or condition.

Seventh character S, sequela, is for use for complications or conditions that arise as a direct result of a condition, such as scar formation after a burn. The scars are a sequela of the burn. When using seventh character S, it is necessary to use both the injury code that precipitated the sequela and the code for the sequela itself. The S is added only to the injury code, not the sequela code. The seventh character S identifies the injury responsible for the sequela. The specific type of sequela (e.g., scar) is sequenced first, followed by the injury code.

The aftercare Z codes should not be used for aftercare for conditions such as injuries or poisonings, where seventh characters are provided to identify subsequent care. For example, for aftercare of an injury, assign the acute injury code with the seventh character D, subsequent encounter.

There are combination codes for poisonings and the associated external cause (accidental, intentional self-harm, assault, undetermined).

The seventh character in Chapter 15 represents the fetus in a multiple gestation that is affected by the condition being coded. These are discussed in more detail in the Pregnancy, Childbirth and the Puerperium lesson.

## *Chapter 1: Certain infectious and parasitic diseases (A00-B99)*

This chapter of ICD-10-CM covers two alpha-characters, A and B. The following notes are available at the beginning of the chapter:

*Includes*:          Diseases generally recognized as communicable or transmissible

Use additional code to identify resistance to antimicrobial drugs (Z16-)

*Excludes1*:          Certain localized Infections - see body system-related chapters infectious and parasitic diseases complicating pregnancy, childbirth and the puerperium (O98.-) influenza and other acute respiratory infections (J00-J22)

*Excludes2*:          Carrier or suspected carrier of infections disease (Z22.-)
infectious and parasitic diseases specific to the perinatal period (P35-P39)

Chapter 1 of ICD-10-CM includes a new section called infections with a predominantly sexual mode of transmission (A50-A64). Many codes have been moved from other places in the classification to this section.

When coding sepsis or AIDS, it is important to review the coding guidelines and the notes at the category level of ICD-10-CM.

There is an important note in the Sequelae of Infectious and Parasitic Diseases (B90-B94) section. Note: Categories B90-B94 are to be used to indicate conditions in categories A00-B89 as the cause of sequelae, which are themselves classified elsewhere. The "sequelae" include conditions specified as such; they also include residuals of diseases classifiable to the above categories if there is evidence that the disease itself is no longer present. Codes from these categories are not to be used for chronic infections. Code chronic current infections to active infectious disease as appropriate.

Code first condition resulting from (sequela) the infectious or parasitic disease.

Bacterial and viral infectious agents (B95-B97) also have a note that specifies that these categories are provided for use as supplementary or additional codes to identify the infectious agent(s) in diseases classified elsewhere. The following are examples of how to index these conditions:
- Infection, infected, infective; bacterial as cause of disease classified elsewhere; Streptococcus group A – B95.0
- Streptococcus, streptococcal; group A, as cause of disease classified elsewhere – B95.0

## Chapter 1 Coding Cases

**1.1.** This 80-year-old female patient was seen with fever, malaise, and left flank pain. A urinalysis was performed and showed bacteria more than 100,000/ml. This was followed by a culture, showing E. coli growth as the cause of the UTI. What **diagnosis** codes are assigned?

Code(s): _____

---

**Coding Guideline I.C.1.c. Infections Resistant to Antibiotics**
Many bacterial infections are resistant to current antibiotics. It is necessary to identify all infections documented as antibiotic resistant. Assign a code from category Z16, Resistance to antimicrobial drugs, following the infection code only if the infection codes does not identify drug resistance.

---

**1.2.** This 78-year-old gentleman is seen for continued follow-up for C. diff colitis. Cultures of the organism have found this infection to be resistant to flagyl. A new drug regimen will be started at this time. What is the correct **diagnosis** code assignment?

Code(s): _____

---

**Coding Guideline I.B.10. Sequela (Late Effects)**
A *sequela* is the residual effect (condition produced) after the acute phase of an illness or injury has terminated. There is no time limit on when a sequela code can be used. The residual may be apparent early, such as in cerebral infarction, or it may occur months or years later, such as that due to a previous injury. Coding of sequela generally requires two codes sequenced in the following order: The condition or nature of the sequela is sequenced first. The sequela code is sequenced second.

---

**1.3.** This patient is seen for right lower leg muscle atrophy as a result of a previous bout of polio. What **diagnosis** codes are assigned?

Code(s): _____

**1.4.** This patient is seen for an acute case of bacterial food poisoning due to Salmonella. No complications are present at this time and the patient will be treated appropriately. What **diagnosis** codes are assigned?

Code(s): _____

---

**Coding Note:** ICD-10-CM has created a range of codes to identify infections with a predominantly sexual mode of transmission (A50-A64). It is important to note that human immunodeficiency virus [HIV] disease is excluded from this range of codes.

**1.5.** This young woman is seen for pelvic pain due to pelvic inflammatory disease. The source of the PID is a result of sexually transmitted chlamydia. What **diagnosis** codes are assigned?

Code(s): _____

---

**Coding Guideline I.C.1.a.2.a. Patient Admitted for HIV-related Condition**
If a patient is admitted with an HIV-related condition, the principal diagnosis should be B20, Human immunodeficiency virus [HIV] disease followed by additional diagnosis codes for all reported HIV-related conditions.

---

**1.6.** This 42-year-old HIV positive male has a fever and shortness of breath. The diagnostic workup, including chest x-ray and sputum culture, resulted in a diagnosis of Pneumocystis pneumonia. This was documented as Pneumocystis pneumonia due to AIDS. What **diagnosis** codes are assigned?

Code(s): _____

---

**Coding Guideline I.C.1.d.1.a. Sepsis**
For a diagnosis of sepsis, assign the appropriate code for the underlying systemic infection. If the type of infection or causal organism is not further specified, assign code A41.9, Sepsis, unspecified organism.

A code from subcategory R65.2, Severe sepsis, should not be assigned unless severe sepsis or an associated acute organ dysfunction is documented.

---

**1.7.** This 87-year-old nursing home patient is being treated with IV antibiotics for E. coli sepsis. What **diagnosis** codes are assigned?

Code(s): _____

---

**Coding Guideline I.C.1.d.1.b. Severe Sepsis**
The coding of severe sepsis requires a minimum of two codes: first a code for the underlying systemic infection, followed by a code from subcategory R65.2, Severe sepsis. If the causal organism is not documented, assign code A41.9, Sepsis, unspecified organism, for the infection. Additional code(s) for the associated organ dysfunction are also required.

---

**1.8.** This 75-year-old woman was taken to the emergency department after being found semi-conscious with markedly abnormal vital signs, a fever of over 39 degrees C, a heart rate of 100, and a respiratory rate of 22/min. On admission to the ICU the physician documented her condition as severe sepsis with acute respiratory failure. The final diagnosis, provided by the physician, was gram-negative sepsis with acute respiratory failure. What **diagnosis** codes are assigned?

Code(s): _____

> **Coding Guideline I.C.1.d.2. Septic Shock**
>
> Septic shock generally refers to circulatory failure associated with severe sepsis and, therefore, it represents a type of acute organ dysfunction.
>
> For cases of septic shock, the code for the systemic infection should be sequenced first, followed by code R65.21, Severe sepsis with septic shock or code T81.12, Postprocedural septic shock. Any additional codes for the other acute organ dysfunctions should also be assigned. As noted in the sequencing instructions in the Tabular List, the code for septic shock cannot be assigned as a principal diagnosis.

**1.9.**   This 25-year-old woman was transferred from an outside facility for treatment of septic shock and acute meningococcal sepsis. The outside facility was unable to manage her severe illness. What **diagnosis** codes are assigned?

Code(s): _____

**1.10.**   This 28-year-old man was admitted with flank pain and renal colic. After diagnostic workup, he was found to have nephrolithiasis. He wanted to avoid surgery and was treated conservatively with fluids and straining of the urine. Two days after admission he developed a cough and fever and was diagnosed with hospital-acquired Pseudomonas pneumonia and was treated appropriately with antibiotics. What **diagnosis** codes are assigned?

Code(s): _____

**1.11.**   This 40-year-old woman with known chronic viral hepatitis resulting from hepatitis B is seen for initiation of antiviral therapy. What **diagnosis** codes are assigned?

Code(s): _____

# Chapter 2: Neoplasms (C00-D49)

All neoplasms are classified in this chapter, whether they are functionally active or not. An additional code from Chapter 4 may be used to identify functional activity associated with any neoplasm.

There have been some changes in the classification system regarding neoplasm coding. A few are listed here:

- Codes moved from other chapters to Chapter 2, for example, Waldenström's macroglobulinemia
- Heading changes, for example, Malignant neoplasm of retroperitoneum and peritoneum moved from Malignant neoplasms of digestive organs and peritoneum to Malignant neoplasms of mesothelial and soft tissue
- Melanoma in situ has a unique category, D03 (previously included in ICD-9-CM category 172, Malignant melanoma of skin)

Neoplasms of uncertain behavior are defined as those whose histologic confirmation whether the neoplasm is malignant or benign cannot be made. Neoplasms of unspecified behavior includes terms such as "growth" NOS, neoplasm NOS, new growth NOS, or tumor NOS. The term "mass," unless otherwise stated, is not to be regarded as a neoplastic growth.

Malignant neoplasms of ectopic tissue are to be coded to the site mentioned; for example, ectopic pancreatic malignant neoplasms are coded to pancreas, unspecified (C25.9).

In addition, notes and coding guidelines govern the correct assignment of codes in this chapter, and should be reviewed.

## Morphology [Histology]

Chapter 2 classifies neoplasms primarily by site (topography), with broad groupings for behavior (malignant, in situ, benign, and so on). The Neoplasm Table should be used to identify the correct topography code. In a few cases, such as for malignant melanoma and certain neuroendocrine tumors, the morphology (histologic type) is included in the category and codes.

---

**Coding Guideline I.C.2. General Neoplasm Guidelines**
The neoplasm table in the Alphabetic Index should be referenced first. However, if the "histological" is documented, that term should be referenced first, rather than going immediately to the Neoplasm Table, in order to determine which column in the Neoplasm Table is appropriate.

---

## Primary Malignant Neoplasms Overlapping Site Boundaries

A primary malignant neoplasm that overlaps two or more contiguous (next to each other) sites should be classified to the subcategory/code .8 (overlapping lesion), unless the combination is specifically indexed elsewhere. For multiple neoplasms of the same site that are not contiguous, such as tumors in different quadrants of the same breast, codes for each site should be assigned.

## Malignant Neoplasm of Ectopic Tissue

Malignant neoplasms of ectopic tissue are to be coded to the site mentioned; for example, ectopic pancreatic malignant neoplasms are coded to pancreas, unspecified (C25.9).

## Chapter 2 Coding Cases

**1.12.** The diagnosis for this 61-year-old female patient is small cell carcinoma of the right lower lobe of the lung with metastasis to the intrathoracic lymph nodes, brain, and right rib. What **diagnosis** codes are assigned?

Code(s): _____

**1.13.** Assign the code(s) for the following diagnosis: Benign carcinoid of the cecum.

Code(s): _____

**1.14.** Assign the code(s) for the following diagnosis: Subacute monocytic leukemia in remission.

Code(s): _____

**1.15.** This 25-year-old female is treated for melanoma of the left breast and left arm. What **diagnosis** codes are assigned?

Code(s): _____

---

**Coding Guideline I.C.2.c.3. Management of Dehydration Due to the Malignancy**
When the admission/encounter is for management of dehydration due to the malignancy or the therapy, or a combination of both, and only the dehydration is being treated (Intravenous rehydration), the dehydration is sequenced first, followed by the code(s) for the malignancy.

---

**Coding Guideline I.C.6.b.5. Neoplasm-Related Pain**
Code G89.3 is assigned to pain documented as being related, associated, or due to cancer, primary or secondary malignancy, or tumor. The code is assigned regardless of whether the pain is acute or chronic.

This code may be assigned as the principal or first-listed code when the stated reason for the admission/encounter is documented as pain control/pain management. The underlying neoplasm should be reported as an additional diagnosis.

When the reason for the admission/encounter is management of the neoplasm and the pain associated with the neoplasm is also documented, code G89.3 may be assigned as an additional diagnosis. It is not necessary to assign an additional code for the site of the pain.

---

**1.16.** This female patient with terminal carcinoma of the central portion of the right breast, metastatic to the liver and brain, was seen for dehydration and chronic intractable neoplasm-related pain. Patient was rehydrated with IVs and given IV pain medication with no treatment directed toward the cancer. What **diagnosis** codes are assigned?

Code(s): _____

**1.17.** This 50-year-old female was diagnosed with left breast carcinoma four years ago, at which time she had a left mastectomy performed with chemotherapy administration. She has been well since that time with no further treatment except for yearly checkups. The patient is now being seen with visual disturbances, dizziness, headaches, and blurred vision. Workup was completed which revealed metastasis to the brain, accounting for these symptoms. This was identified as being metastatic from the breast, not a new primary. What **diagnosis** codes are assigned?

Code(s): _____

---

**Coding Guideline I.C.2.e.2. Patient Admission/Encounter Solely for Administration of Chemotherapy, Immunotherapy, and Radiation Therapy**

If a patient admission/encounter is solely for the administration of chemotherapy, immunotherapy, or radiation therapy assign code Z51.0, Encounter for antineoplastic radiation therapy; Z51.11, Encounter for antineoplastic chemotherapy; or Z51.12, Encounter of antineoplastic immunotherapy as the first-listed or principal diagnosis. If a patient receives more than one of these therapies during the same admission more than one of these codes may be assigned, in any sequence.

---

**1.18.** The encounter is to receive chemotherapy following the recent diagnosis of carcinoma of the small intestines. The tumor was in the area where the duodenum and jejunum join. The cancer was resected two months ago and the patient has been receiving chemotherapy. What **diagnosis** codes are assigned?

Code(s): _____

# Chapter 3: Diseases of the blood and blood-forming organs and certain disorders involving the immune mechanism (D50-D89)

Chapter 3 of ICD-10-CM includes codes primarily from ICD-9-CM Chapter 4, Diseases of the Blood and Blood-Forming Organs, but also includes many codes from ICD-9-CM Chapter 3, Endocrine, Nutritional and Metabolic Diseases and Immunity Disorders. It also includes some codes from ICD-9-CM Chapter 1, Infectious and Parasitic Diseases (for example, sarcoidosis).

## Chapter 3 Coding Cases

> **Coding Guideline I.C.2.c.1. Anemia Associated with Malignancy**
> When admission/encounter is for management of an anemia associated with the malignancy, and the treatment is only for anemia, the appropriate code for the malignancy is sequenced as the principal or first-listed diagnosis followed by the appropriate code for the anemia (such as D63.0, Anemia in neoplastic disease).

**1.19.** This elderly woman is receiving a blood transfusion for severe anemia due to her left breast carcinoma. Assign the correct **diagnosis** code(s).

Code(s): _____

**1.20.** Code the following: Congenital red cell aplastic anemia.

Code(s): _____

**1.21.** This patient is seen for continued follow-up regarding his periodic neutropenia. Assign the correct **diagnosis** code(s).

Code(s): _____

**1.22.** Code the following: Thalassemia, minor.

Code(s): _____

**1.23.** This 48-year-old female is seen for sickle-cell crisis with acute chest syndrome. Assign the correct **diagnosis** code(s).

Code(s): _____

**1.24.** Code the following diagnosis: Severe combined immunodeficiency [SCID] with low T- and B-cell numbers.

Code(s): _____

# Chapter 4: Endocrine, nutritional and metabolic diseases (E00-E89)

All neoplasms, whether functionally active or not, are classified in Chapter 2. Appropriate codes in Chapter 4 (namely, E05.8, E07.0, E16-E31, E34.-) may be used as additional codes to indicate either functional activity by neoplasms and ectopic endocrine tissue or hyperfunction and hypofunction of endocrine glands associated with neoplasms and other conditions classified elsewhere. Excluded in this chapter are transitory endocrine and metabolic disorders specific to the newborn (P70-P74).

### Diabetes Mellitus

The diabetes mellitus codes are now combination codes that include the type of diabetes, the body system affected, and the complications affecting that body system. As many diabetes codes as are necessary to describe all of the complications of the disease may be used, and should be sequenced based on the reason for a particular encounter. The diabetes mellitus codes are no longer classified as controlled or uncontrolled. There is a note in the Index that inadequately controlled, out of control, and poorly controlled are coded to Diabetes, by type, with hyperglycemia.

The categories for diabetes in ICD-10-CM are
- Diabetes mellitus due to underlying condition (E08)
- Drug or chemical induced diabetes mellitus (E09)
- Type 1 diabetes mellitus (E10)
- Type 2 diabetes mellitus (E11)
- Other specified diabetes mellitus (E13)

It is important to review the coding guidelines and the notes in each category when coding diabetes mellitus. There is one particular note available in each category except for diabetes mellitus type 1. This note states "Use additional code to identify any insulin use (Z79.4)." This code would not be assigned with type 1 cases because insulin is required to sustain life.

## Chapter 4 Coding Cases

**Coding Guideline I.C.4.a. Diabetes Mellitus**
The diabetes mellitus codes are combination codes that include the type of diabetes mellitus, the body system affected, and the complications affecting that body system. As many codes within a particular category as are necessary to describe all of the complications of the disease may be used. They should be sequenced based on the reason for a particular encounter. Assign as many codes from categories E08-E13 as needed to identify all of the associated conditions that the patient has.

**1.25.** This 62-year-old male is being seen for mild nonproliferative diabetic retinopathy with macular edema. He has type 2 DM and takes insulin on a daily basis. He also has diabetic cataract in his right eye. What **diagnosis** codes are assigned?

Code(s): _____

**1.26.** The patient, a type 1 diabetic with diabetic chronic kidney disease, stage 3, is being seen for regulation of insulin dosage. The patient has an abscessed right molar, which was determined, in part, to be responsible for elevation of the patient's blood sugar. What **diagnosis** codes are assigned?

Code(s): _____

**Coding Guideline I.C.4.a.6. Secondary Diabetes Mellitus**
Codes under categories E08, Diabetes mellitus due to underlying condition, and E09, Drug or chemical induced diabetes mellitus, identify complications/manifestations associated with secondary diabetes mellitus. Secondary diabetes is always caused by another condition or event (e.g., cystic fibrosis, malignant neoplasm of pancreas, pancreatectomy, adverse effect of drug, poisoning).

**Coding Guideline I.C.4.a.6.b. Assigning and Sequencing Secondary Diabetes Codes and Its Causes**
The sequencing of the secondary diabetes codes in relationship to codes for the cause of the diabetes is based on the Tabular List instructions for categories E08 and E09.

**1.27.** Assign the codes for a 32-year-old female with secondary diabetes mellitus due to acute idiopathic pancreatitis. She has diabetic hyperglycemia and takes insulin.

Code(s): _____

**1.28.** Assign the code(s) for the following diagnosis: Morbid obesity with a BMI of 42 in an adult.

Code(s): _____

**1.29.** Assign the code(s) for the following diagnosis: Bulimia with moderate protein–calorie malnutrition.

Code(s): _____

**1.30.** The patient was seen with severe abdominal cramping, nausea and vomiting, and diarrhea. She states that she ate turkey salad several hours before these symptoms developed. The patient has had the symptoms for about 15 hours. Lab tests show dehydration. The patient was treated with IV therapy. Diagnosis: Dehydration. Salmonella gastroenteritis, abdominal cramping, nausea, vomiting, and diarrhea. What **diagnosis** codes are assigned?

Code(s): _____

**1.31.** The patient is a 31-year-old male with a history of type 1 diabetes mellitus and is on 15 units of NPH and 10 units of Regular in the morning, and 10 units of NPH and 5 of Regular in the evening. The patient is currently having symptoms of nausea with severe vomiting. The patient at the same time has had increased frequency of urination and polydipsia. The patient is also severely dehydrated. The patient was hydrated, and, as a result, his blood sugar decreased from more than 600 to normal levels. The patient was diagnosed with diabetic ketoacidosis, type 1. What **diagnosis** codes are assigned?

Code(s): _____

---

**Coding Guideline I.C.19.e.5.a. Adverse Effect**
When coding an adverse effect of a drug that has been correctly prescribed and properly administered, assign the appropriate code for the nature of the adverse effect followed by the appropriate code for the adverse effect of the drug (T36-T50). The code for the drug should have a fifth or sixth character 5.

---

**Coding Note:** A note appears in the Tabular, under category E09, instructing to "Use additional code for adverse effect, if applicable, to identify drug (T36-T50 with fifth or sixth character 5)." **Use the Drugs and Chemical Table to locate this code.**

An additional note appears in the Tabular under category E09 instructing to "Use additional code to identify any insulin use (Z79.4)."

---

**1.32.** The 34-year-old patient is being seen for ongoing management of steroid-induced diabetes mellitus which was due to the prolonged use of corticosteroids, which have been discontinued. The patient's diabetes is managed with insulin which he has been taking for the last two years. What **diagnosis** codes are assigned?

Code(s): _____

**1.33.** The patient is being seen because of increasingly irritating symptomatology, including nervousness, irritability, increased perspiration, shakiness and increased appetite with unexplained weight loss, increased heart rate, palpitations, and sleeping difficulties. A thyroid stimulating hormone test revealed elevated levels and a thyroid nuclear medicine scan revealed hyperactivity of the entire thyroid gland. Based on the diagnostic findings the patient was diagnosed with hyperthyroidism with multinodular goiter. The patient was started on oral anti-thyroid medication. Arrangements were also made for patient to see a cardiologist due to the fact that her palpitations were more pronounced than seen in other patients with hyperthyroidism. What **diagnosis** codes are assigned?

Code(s): _____

**1.34.** This type 1 diabetic patient has a severe chronic diabetic left foot ulcer with diabetic peripheral angiopathy. He also has diabetic stage 2 chronic kidney disease. He is being evaluated to see if debridement is required for this ulcer with breakdown of the skin. What **diagnosis** codes are assigned?

Code(s): _____

## Chapter 5: Mental, behavioral and neurodevelopmental disorders (F01-F99)

The codes in this chapter include disorders of psychological development, but exclude symptoms, signs, and abnormal clinical laboratory finding (R00-R99). The arrangement of the codes within the various sections of ICD-10-CM is significantly different.

A number of changes to category and subcategory titles have been made; for example, ICD-9-CM subcategory 296.0 is Bipolar I disorder, single manic episode, but the ICD-10-CM counterpart, category F30, is Manic episode.

There are unique codes for alcohol and drug use (not specified as abuse or dependence), and abuse and dependence, so careful review of the documentation is required. And there are changes to the codes for drug and alcohol abuse and dependence as they no longer identify continuous or episodic use. A history of drug or alcohol dependence is coded as "in remission." Further, there are combination codes for drug and alcohol use and associated conditions, such as withdrawal, sleep disorders, or psychosis. There is a code for blood alcohol level (Y90.-) that can be assigned as an additional code when documentation indicates its use.

There is a change in sequencing involving the intellectual disability codes (F70-F79). In ICD-9-CM, an additional code for any associated psychiatric or physical condition(s) should be sequenced after the intellectual disability code. In ICD-10-CM, any associated physical or developmental disorder should be coded first.

### Chapter 5 Coding Cases

**1.35.** Code the following diagnosis: Alcohol abuse with intoxication.

Code(s): _____

**1.36.** This young man is seen for continued follow-up for treatment of his dependence on amphetamines. How should this diagnosis be coded?

Code(s): _____

**1.37.** This 25-year-old male presents to the clinic requesting assistance for cessation of chewing tobacco use. He has been a chronic user of chewing tobacco since age 13 and is now motivated to quit. Counseling on the options for chewing tobacco cessation was provided to the patient. Diagnosis: Counseling for cessation of tobacco dependence. What **diagnosis** codes are assigned?

Code(s): _____

**Coding Note:** The ICD-10-CM classification system does not provide separate "history" codes for alcohol and drug abuse. These conditions are identified as "in remission" in ICD-10-CM.

**Coding Guideline I.C.5.b.1. In Remission**
Selection of codes for "in remission" for categories F10-F19, Mental and behavioral disorders due to psychoactive substance use (categories F10-F19 with -.21) requires the provider's clinical judgment. The appropriate codes for "in remission" are assigned only on the basis of provider documentation (as defined in the Official Guidelines for Coding and Reporting).

**1.38.**   Joe, a 43-year-old male, is currently receiving treatment for alcohol dependence. As a result of Joe's drinking he is also on medication for chronic alcoholic gastritis. He also has a history of cocaine dependence. What **diagnosis** codes are assigned?

Code(s): _____

**1.39.**   The patient is seen for individual psychotherapy as part of his long-term treatment for borderline personality disorder. His condition is described as "cluster B personality disorder." The patient has been taking his monoamine oxidase inhibitor (MAOI) medication and reports he feels it has helped him manage his impulsive, overly emotional, and erratic behavior. The patient is also a recovering alcoholic which the therapist describes as being "in remission." The patient will return next week for his scheduled appointment. What **diagnosis** codes are assigned?

Code(s): _____

**Coding Note:** ICD-10-CM provides a code to indicate blood alcohol level. Under the category F10, there is a "use additional code" note for blood alcohol level. Blood alcohol level can be indexed in the Index to External Causes.

**1.40.**   This 18-year-old male has been drinking since he was 13. He was brought to the ER and then admitted because of acute alcohol inebriation. Blood alcohol level shows 22 mg/100 ml. The discharge diagnosis is acute alcohol intoxication with chronic alcohol dependence, continuous. What **diagnosis** codes are assigned?

Code(s): _____

# Chapter 6: Diseases of the nervous system (G00-G99)

Sense organs have been separated from nervous system disorders, creating two new chapters for diseases of eye and adnexa (Chapter 7) and diseases of the ear and mastoid process (Chapter 8).

The following conditions have been moved from ICD-9-CM Chapter 7: Diseases of the Circulatory System, to ICD-10-CM Chapter 6: Basilar and carotid artery syndromes, transient global amnesia, and transient cerebral ischemic attack.

A note at categories G81 (Hemiplegia and hemiparesis), G82 (Paraplegia and quadriplegia) and G83 (Other paralytic syndromes) provides this information: This category is to be used only when the listed conditions are reported without further specification, or are stated to be old or longstanding but of unspecified cause. The category is also for use in multiple coding to identify these conditions resulting from any cause. Paralytic sequelae of cerebral infarct/stroke are in Chapter 9: Diseases of the circulatory system.

The terminology for epilepsy has been updated, with terms to classify the disorder such as: localization-related idiopathic epilepsy, generalized idiopathic epilepsy, and special epileptic syndromes. Within those various categories, more specificity is possible, such as identifying seizures of localized onset, complex partial seizures, intractable, and status epilepticus. A note with category G40, Epilepsy and recurrent seizures and G43, Migraine provides the following terms to be considered equivalent to intractable: pharmacoresistent (pharmacologically resistant), treatment resistant, refractory (medically), and poorly controlled.

## Chapter 6 Coding Cases

**1.41.** This 52-year-old male has been having increasing dementia and forgetfulness. He has been wandering off and leaving his home and forgetting where he is or where he is going. The diagnosis of dementia due to early-onset Alzheimer's was established. What **diagnosis** codes are assigned?

Code(s): _____

**1.42.** This patient, a 15-year-old female, is being seen for management of juvenile myoclonic epilepsy. The patient did not respond to treatment and was diagnosed with an intractable seizure. What **diagnosis** codes are assigned?

Code(s): _____

> **Coding Guideline I.C.6.a. Dominant/Nondominant Side**
> Codes from category G81, Hemiplegia and hemiparesis, and subcategories, G83.1, Monoplegia of lower limb, G83.2, Monoplegia of upper limb, and G83.3, Monoplegia, unspecified, identify whether the dominant or nondominant side is affected. Should the affected side be documented, but not specified as dominant or nondominant and the classification system does not indicate a default, code selection is as follows:
> - For ambidextrous patients, the default should be dominant
> - If the left side is affected the default is nondominant
> - If the right side is affected the default is dominant

**1.43.** Assign the code(s) for the following diagnosis: Left-sided hemiplegia.

Code(s): _____

> **Coding Guideline II.C. Two or More Diagnoses that Equally Meet the Definition of Principal Diagnosis**
> In the unusual instance when two or more diagnoses equally meet the criteria for principal diagnosis as determined by the circumstances of admission, diagnostic workup, and/or therapy provided, and the Alphabetic Index, Tabular List, or another coding guideline does not provide sequencing direction, any one of the diagnoses may be sequenced first.

**1.44.** The patient was admitted with high fever, stiff neck, chest pain, and nausea. A lumbar puncture was performed and results were positive for meningitis. Chest x-ray revealed pneumonia. Sputum cultures grew pneumococcus. Patient was treated with IV antibiotics. The established diagnoses were pneumococcal meningitis and pneumococcal pneumonia. Code the **diagnoses** for this case only.

Code(s): _____

**1.45.** This patient has been taking Haloperidol as prescribed for paranoid schizophrenia. He is being seen for change in facial expressions and stiffness in the arms and legs. Diagnosis: Secondary Parkinsonism due to Haloperidol. The drug will be discontinued. What **diagnosis** codes are assigned?

Code(s): _____

**1.46.** This 45-year-old female patient has breast cancer of the right breast with multiple metastases to the liver. She is seen to control the severe acute pain of the liver metastases. What **diagnosis** codes are assigned?

Code(s): _____

**1.47.** The patient, a type 2 diabetic with neuropathy, developed weakness of the left arm and leg. The patient was brought to the emergency room where he could speak but was unable to use his left arm and leg. Diagnostic radiographic procedures were scheduled; however, the patient completely recovered and was able to ambulate with no neurological deficits within 24 hours. Due to the complete recovery, it was determined that the patient had experienced a TIA. During this encounter the patient also was treated for an intractable classical migraine. What **diagnosis** codes are assigned?

Code(s): _____

# Chapter 7: Diseases of the eye and adnexa (H00-H59)

Chapter 7 is a new chapter in ICD-10-CM, and these conditions were previously included with Diseases of the Nervous System and Sense Organs.

Codes have been expanded to increase anatomic specificity and add the concept of laterality. Many of the codes include right, left, bilateral, and unspecified eye. If the option of bilateral is not available (e.g., eczematous dermatitis of eyelid), and the condition is present in both eyes, it is correct to assign the code for right and left. If, however, a code exists for bilateral, that should be assigned, not right and left eye.

## Chapter 7 Coding Cases

**1.48.** This 40-year-old woman presents to her physician with bilateral eye pain. Her condition is diagnosed as nonulcerative bilateral blepharitis of the upper eyelids. What is the correct **diagnosis** coding for this case?

Code(s): _____

**1.49.** Code the following diagnosis: Recurrent pterygium, bilateral.

Code(s): _____

**1.50.** This elderly woman is seen in the clinic for follow-up of her age-related nuclear cataract. At this time, it is only in her left eye. Code the **diagnosis** for this case.

Code(s): _____

> **Coding Note:** Multiple codes in the H40 category require a seventh character to designate the stage of the glaucoma. These stages are as follows:
>
> 0 – stage unspecified
> 1 – mild stage
> 2 – moderate stage
> 3 – severe stage
> 4 – indeterminate stage

> **Coding Guideline I.C.7.a.5. Indeterminate Stage Glaucoma**
> Assignment of the seventh character 4, Indeterminate stage, should be based on the clinical documentation. The seventh character 4 is used for glaucomas whose stage cannot be clinically determined. This seventh character should not be confused with the seventh character 0, unspecified, which should be assigned when there is no documentation regarding the stage of the glaucoma.

**1.51.** This is a visit for this patient with moderate primary open-angle glaucoma of the left eye. What is the correct **diagnosis** code for this case?

Code(s): _____

**1.52.** This patient presents to his physician with continued eye problems following cataract surgery. Ultimately, this is diagnosed as bullous keratopathy, left eye, due to cataract surgery. What is the correct **diagnosis** codes?

Code(s): _____

**1.53.** This elderly woman was being treated for her right eye age-related cortical cataract at this day-surgery center. After the procedure was completed, the patient suffered a postoperative hemorrhage of the eye. This was addressed by the surgeon. What is the correct **diagnosis** code(s)?

Code(s): _____

## *Chapter 8: Diseases of the ear and mastoid process (H60-H95)*

Chapter 8 is also a new chapter in ICD-10-CM and includes conditions previously found in the Nervous System and Sense Organs chapter.

Codes have also been expanded to increase anatomic specificity and add the concept of laterality.

A number of new instructional notes have been added. The note at the beginning of the chapter states to use an external cause code following the code for the ear condition, if applicable, to identify the cause of the ear condition.

The following note addresses otitis media categories H65, H66:
> Use additional code for any associated perforated tympanic membrane (H72.-)
> Use additional code to identify:
>> exposure to environmental tobacco smoke (Z77.22)
>> exposure to tobacco smoke in the perinatal period (P96.81)
>> history of tobacco use (Z87.891)
>> occupational exposure to environmental tobacco smoke (Z57.31)
>> tobacco dependence (F17.-)
>> tobacco use (Z72.0)

Notes indicating that the underlying disease should be coded first have been added; for example, there is a note under the ICD-10-CM category for perforation of tympanic membrane indicating that any associated otitis media should be coded first.

### *Chapter 8 Coding Cases*

**1.54.** A five-year-old female is seen for acute ear pain. Examination reveals left acute serous otitis media. Further examination revealed a total perforated tympanic membrane of the right ear due to chronic otitis media. What **diagnoses** codes are assigned?

Code(s): _____

**1.55.** Assign the code for the following diagnosis: Ménière's vertigo of left ear.

Code(s): _____

**1.56.** This 50-year-old female, admitted to the hospital for surgery, has bilateral conductive hearing loss due to nonobliterative otosclerosis of the stapes at the oval window. She is unable to hear with hearing aids and has decided to undergo left stapedectomy. During the surgery an inadvertent laceration was made to the tympanic meatal flap, which was repaired. What **diagnosis** codes are assigned?

Code(s): _____

# Chapter 9: Diseases of the circulatory system (I00-I99)

Some codes have been moved to Chapter 9 from other chapters in ICD-9-CM, for example, Binswanger's disease; chronic and mesenteric lymphadenitis; and gangrene.

The type of hypertension (benign, malignant, unspecified) is not used as an axis for the ICD-10-CM hypertension codes; there is only one code for essential hypertension (I10).

The category for late effects of cerebrovascular disease has been retitled "Sequelae of cerebrovascular disease," and it has been restructured by expanding all subcategory codes. This expansion involves specifying laterality, changing subcategory titles, making terminology changes, adding sixth characters, and providing greater specificity in general. Late effects of cerebrovascular disease are differentiated by type of stroke (hemorrhage, infarction).

The terminology has changed for some cardiovascular conditions; for example, "intermediate coronary syndrome" has been retitled "unstable angina."

## Acute Myocardial Infarction (AMI)

The time frame for acute myocardial infarction (AMI) codes has changed from eight weeks or less in ICD-9-CM to four weeks or less in ICD-10-CM.

In the acute myocardial infarction codes, ST elevation (STEMI) and non-ST elevation (NSTEMI) are in the ICD-10-CM code titles instead of just being inclusion terms.

Chapter 9 contains codes for initial AMIs (I21) and subsequent AMIs (I22). A code from category I22, Subsequent ST elevation (STEMI) and non-ST elevation (NSTEMI) myocardial infarction is to be used when a patient who has suffered an AMI has a new AMI within the four-week time frame of the initial AMI. A code from category I22 must be used in conjunction with a code from category I21. The sequencing of the I22 and I21 codes depends on the circumstances of the encounter.

It is important to review the use additional code related to tobacco use or exposure.

## Chapter 9 Coding Cases

**1.57.** This patient is seen today for follow-up for his benign hypertension. What is the correct **diagnosis** code?

Code(s): _____

> **Coding Guideline I.C.9.a.3. Hypertensive Heart and Chronic Kidney Disease**
> Assign codes from combination category I13, Hypertensive heart and chronic kidney disease, when both hypertensive kidney disease and hypertensive heart disease are stated in the diagnosis. Assume a relationship between the hypertension and the chronic kidney disease, whether or not the condition is so designated. If heart failure is present, assign an additional code from category I50 to identify the type of heart failure.
>
> The appropriate code from category N18, Chronic kidney disease, should be used as a secondary code with a code from I13 to identify the stage of chronic kidney disease.

**1.58.** Code the following diagnoses: Stage 3 chronic kidney disease with congestive heart failure (CHF) due to hypertension.

Code(s): _____

> **Coding Guideline I.C.9.e.3. AMI Documented as Nontransmural or Subendocardial but Site Provided**
> If an AMI is documented as nontransmural or subendocardial, but the site is provided, it is still coded as subendocardial AMI.

> **Coding Guideline I.C.9.e.1. ST Elevation Myocardial Infarction (STEMI) and Non-ST Elevation Myocardial Infarction (NSTEMI)**
> If NSTEMI evolves to STEMI, assign the STEMI code. If STEMI converts to NSTEMI due to thrombolytic therapy, it is still coded as a STEMI.

**1.59.** This 54-year-old female is being treated for an acute non-ST anterior wall myocardial infarction which she suffered 5 days ago. She also has atrial fibrillation. What is the correct **diagnosis** code(s)?

Code(s): _____

> **Coding Guideline I.C.9.e.4. Subsequent Myocardial Infarction**
> A code from category I22, Subsequent ST elevation (STEMI) and non-ST elevation (NSTEMI) myocardial infarction is to be used when a patient who has suffered an AMI has a new AMI within the 4 week time frame of the initial AMI. A code from category I22 must be used in conjunction with a code from category I21. The sequencing of the I22 and I21 codes depends on the circumstances of the encounter.

**1.60.** This same patient (from problem #1.59) presented to the emergency department two weeks later and was diagnosed with an acute inferior wall myocardial infarction. She is still being monitored following her initial heart attack two weeks earlier and continues to have atrial fibrillation. She will be transferred to a larger facility for cardiac catheterization and possible further intervention. What **diagnosis** codes are assigned?

Code(s): _____

> **Coding Note:** A code from category I23 must be used in conjunction with a code from category I21 or category I22. The I23 code should be sequenced first, if it is the reason for encounter, or, it should be sequenced after the I21 or I22 code if the complication of the MI occurs during the encounter for the MI.

**1.61.** This patient is seen in consultation after readmission for postinfarction angina. She was discharged two days ago after treatment for an anterior wall ST elevation myocardial infarction. What is the correct **diagnosis** code assignment?

Code(s): _____

> **Coding Guideline I.C.9.b. Atherosclerotic Coronary Artery Disease and Angina**
> ICD-10-CM has combination codes for atherosclerotic heart disease with angina pectoris. The subcategories for these codes are I25.11, Atherosclerotic heart disease of native coronary artery with angina pectoris and I25.7, Atherosclerosis of coronary artery bypass graft(s) and coronary artery of transplanted heart with angina pectoris.
>
> When using one of these combination codes it is not necessary to use an additional code for angina pectoris. A causal relationship can be assumed in a patient with both atherosclerosis and angina pectoris, unless the documentation indicates the angina is due to something other than the atherosclerosis.

**1.62.** What is the correct **diagnosis** coding for a patient with coronary artery disease (CAD) with angina? This patient has no previous history of CABG.

Code(s): _____

**1.63.** This 63-year-old male is being seen for treatment of his unstable angina. This gentleman has a history of 2-vessel coronary artery bypass approximately 18 months ago. A recent cardiac catheterization shows continued evidence of coronary arteriosclerosis but both of the bypass grafts are patent. Also, of note, is that this patient suffered a cerebrovascular infarction three years ago which resulted in right-side (dominant) hemiparesis. What is the correct diagnosis code(s)?

Code(s): _____

**1.64.** This 75-year-old man is seen today for treatment of his congestive heart failure. After study, the final **diagnosis** was documented as acute on chronic diastolic congestive heart failure. What is the correct diagnosis code assignment?

Code(s): _____

**1.65.** Code the following case: Acute cerebral infarction, thrombosis of the left anterior cerebral artery with residual right-sided hemiplegia.

Code(s): _____

> **Coding Guideline I.C.9.d.1. Category I69, Sequelae of Cerebrovascular Disease**
> Category I69 is used to indicate conditions classifiable to categories I60-I67 as the causes of sequela (neurologic deficits), themselves classified elsewhere. These "late effects" include neurologic deficits that persist after the initial onset of conditions classifiable to categories I60-I67. The neurologic deficits caused by cerebrovascular disease may be present from the onset or may arise at any time after the onset of the condition classifiable to categories I60-I67.
>
> Codes from category I69, Sequelae of cerebrovascular disease, that specify hemiplegia, hemiparesis and monoplegia identify whether the dominant or nondominant side is affected. Should the affected side be documented, but not specified as dominant or nondominant, and the classification system does not indicate a default, code selection is as follows:
> For ambidextrous patients, the default should be dominant
> If the left side is affected, the default is non-dominant
> If the right side is affected, the default is dominant

> **Coding Guideline I.C.9.d.2. Codes from Category I69 with Codes from I60-I67**
> Codes from category I69 may be assigned on a health care record with codes from I60-I67, if the patient has a current cerebrovascular disease and deficits from an old cerebrovascular disease.

**1.66.** This pleasant gentleman is seen in the clinic to follow up from a previous stroke. He suffered a cerebrovascular infarction 6 months ago which left him with aphasia and left-sided hemiparesis on his nondominant side. The patient will be referred to outpatient rehabilitation for speech, physical, and occupational therapy. What is the correct **diagnosis** code(s)?

Code(s): _____

**1.67.** This 62-year-old male patient was admitted to the hospital with progressive episodes of chest pain determined to be crescendo angina. The patient has no previous history of CABG. He had myocardial infarction five years ago and was diagnosed with coronary artery disease and progressively has been having more frequent episodes of chest pain. During the hospital stay, he was given IV nitroglycerin and was subsequently placed on Cardizem for further treatment of his angina. He was scheduled for cardiac catheterization next week. No other complications arose during the hospitalization. What is the correct **diagnosis** code(s)?

Code(s): _____

**1.68.** This patient is seen for evaluation of his continuing unstable angina. After significant evaluation, his symptoms were found to be due to atherosclerosis of his bypassed graft. This is an autologous arterial graft. Final diagnosis: CAD of bypass graft with unstable angina and hypertensive congestive heart failure. The patient will be scheduled for surgery. What is the correct **diagnosis** code(s)?

Code(s): _____

**1.69.** This patient is being treated for a current inferolateral ST elevation myocardial infarction. This case is complicated by the development a hemopericardium as a result of the infarction. What is the correct **diagnosis** code(s)?

Code(s): _____

**1.70.** Assign the correct **diagnosis** code(s): Acute cerebrovascular infarction—embolism of the left cerebellar artery with dysphagia and right hemiplegia.

Code(s): _____

# Chapter 10: Diseases of the respiratory system (J00-J99)

Certain codes have moved to Chapter 10 from other locations, for example, streptococcal sore throat.

Lobar pneumonia has a unique code in a category for pneumonia, unspecified organism, rather than being classified to the code for pneumococcal pneumonia.

The terminology used to describe asthma has been updated to reflect the current clinical classification of asthma. The following terms have been added to describe asthma: mild intermittent and three degrees of persistent—mild persistent, moderate persistent, and severe persistent. Intrinsic asthma (nonallergic) and extrinsic (allergic) are both classified to J45.909, Unspecified asthma, uncomplicated.

A note at the beginning of the chapter states: When a respiratory condition is described as occurring in more than one site and is not specifically indexed, it should be classified to the lower anatomic site (for example, tracheobronchitis to bronchitis in J40).

Some of the codes in Chapter 10 have been expanded to include notes indicating that an additional code should be assigned or an associated condition should be sequenced first. The following are examples of the notations:
- Use additional code to identify the infectious agent
- Use additional code to identify the virus
- Code first any associated lung abscess
- Code first the underlying disease
- Use additional code to identify other conditions such as tobacco use or exposure

### Chapter 10 Coding Cases

**1.71.** A four-year-old child was seen with a high fever, cough, and chest pain. Diagnosis of diffuse bronchopneumonia was made. Gram stain of the sputum showed numerous small gram-negative coccobacilli. Diagnosis: H. influenza pneumonia. What **diagnosis** codes are assigned?

Code(s): _____

**1.72.** The patient has increasing shortness of breath, weakness, and ineffective cough. Treatment included oxygen therapy and advice for smoking cessation. Diagnoses listed as acute respiratory insufficiency due to acute exacerbation of COPD and tobacco dependence. What **diagnosis** codes are assigned?

Code(s): _____

**1.73.** This 10-year-old female child is being seen because of severe persistent asthma with acute exacerbation. What **diagnosis** codes are assigned?

Code(s): _____

**1.74.** This 75-year-old female was brought to the ER with severe difficulty in breathing. She was intubated and started on mechanical ventilation and admitted. Diagnoses for this patient: Acute respiratory failure, acute infectious bronchitis with acute exacerbation of COPD. What **diagnosis** codes are assigned?

Code(s): _____

**1.75.** This 60-year-old male was admitted to the hospital with chest rales, dyspnea, cyanosis, and hypotension. He has severe gastroesophageal reflux causing him to aspirate food. He was treated for his aspiration pneumonia with respiratory therapy and antibiotics. What **diagnosis** codes are assigned?

Code(s): _____

**1.76.** A 17-year-old college student was treated for cough, fever, body aches, and headache. Diagnosis: Upper respiratory tract infection due to novel influenza A virus. What **diagnosis** codes are assigned?

Code(s): _____

**1.77.** The physician has documented the following diagnoses for this elderly patient: COPD with emphysema, CHF, hypertension, and atrial fibrillation. What **diagnosis** codes are assigned?

Code(s): _____

Coding Note: In the Tabular, there is a note under category J44 to code also type of asthma, if applicable (J45.-).

Coding Note: In the Tabular there is an *Excludes2* note under category J45 for asthma with chronic obstructive pulmonary disease.

By definition, when an *Excludes2* note appears under a code, it is acceptable to use both the code and the excluded code together if the patient has both conditions at the same time.

1.78. **Discharge Diagnosis:**

Moderate persistent asthma with status asthmaticus
Acute exacerbation of chronic obstructive pulmonary disease

**Hospital Course:** The patient presented with gradual increase in shortness of breath, which was unresponsive to home nebulizer treatments. In the emergency room, he received more respiratory treatments; however, he failed to improve. Therefore, the patient was admitted to the hospital. At the time of admission, the theophylline level was 5.9. Chest x-ray showed no evidence of active infiltrates. The patient was bolused with intravenous steroids and started on frequent respiratory therapy treatments. IV aminophylline boluses and drip were used to increase his theophylline level to therapeutic range. The patient gradually cleared and by the next day was much better. His IV aminophylline was changed to p.o. The Ventolin treatments were decreased to q 4 hr. and his steroids were rapidly tapered back to 10 mg of Prednisone. What **diagnosis** codes are assigned?

Code(s): _____

1.79. A ventilator-dependent patient (due to COPD with emphysema) is admitted to the hospital for dehydration. IV fluids are started for hydration and the patient is placed on the hospital's ventilator. What is the appropriate **diagnosis** code assignment?

Code(s): _____

Coding Note: A note appears in the Tabular under code I69.391 to use an additional code to identify the type of dysphagia, if known (R13.1-).

1.80. An elderly nursing home patient was seen for pneumonia. The patient has frequent aspiration pneumonia because of his difficulty in swallowing (neurogenic) due to a previous cerebral infarction. In addition to the aspiration-type pneumonia, the patient also has stage 1 decubitus ulcers on both his left and right hip. What **diagnosis** codes are assigned?

Code(s): _____

# Chapter 11: Diseases of the digestive system (K00-K95)

Some of the disease categories in Chapter 11 have been restructured to bring together those groups that are in some way related. For example, Chapter 11 contains two new sections: Diseases of liver (K70-K77) and Disorders of gallbladder, biliary tract, and pancreas (K80-K87). And in some cases, headings of subcategories have been changed; for example, angiodysplasia of intestine is in a subcategory for "other specified disorders of intestine" in ICD-9-CM, whereas it is in a subcategory for "vascular disorders of intestine" in ICD-10-CM.

Instructional notes indicating that an additional code should be assigned for associated conditions and external causes or that an underlying condition should be coded first have been expanded.

## Chapter 11 Coding Cases

**Coding Note:** Hernia with both gangrene and obstruction is classified to hernia with gangrene.

1.81. This patient is seen for treatment of a recurrent right inguinal hernia with gangrene and obstruction. What is the correct code assignment for this case?

Code(s): _____

1.82. Assign the **diagnosis** code(s) for Acute gastric ulcer with hemorrhage.

Code(s): _____

1.83. This patient has been diagnosed with choledocholithiasis with acute cholangitis and obstruction. What is the correct **diagnosis** code(s)?

Code(s): _____

**Coding Note:** ICD-10-CM provides combination codes for complications commonly associated with Crohn's disease. These combination codes can be found under subcategory K50.0.

1.84. This 30-year-old woman has been treated for Crohn's disease of the small intestine since she was 18-years-old. She has had several exacerbations of the disease in the past years. At this time, small bowel x-ray shows a small bowel obstruction. The obstruction was found to be a result of an exacerbation of her Crohn's disease. What is the correct diagnosis code(s)?

Code(s): _____

1.85. A 70-year-old female was visiting relatives in the area and was brought to the emergency department, complaining of vomiting blood and having very dark stools that appeared to be bloody. The patient had gone out to dinner with relatives and shortly after returning home, started vomiting and having diarrhea and blamed it on the large meal. She continued to have these symptoms overnight and her family members insisted she come to the hospital. The patient is taking Prinivil, Lanoxin, and Lasix for congestive heart failure and atrial fibrillation and these medications were continued. The gastroenterologist was called to consult and found a past history of gastric ulcer. The patient had EGD 5 months earlier showing chronic bleeding ulcer in the antrum of the stomach. She was placed on medication and warned that this may be a recurrent problem. The patient refused a follow-up EGD and requested to be released to return home and receive treatment from her regular physician. It should be noted that serial blood counts did not find any significant anemia. The patient was discharged with a diagnosis of chronic bleeding gastric ulcer and copies of her medical records to take home for review by her private physician. What is the correct **diagnosis** code(s)?

Code(s): _____

1.86. A 68-year-old man was admitted to the hospital for bilateral inguinal hernia repair that could not be done on an outpatient basis because of anticipated extended recovery time required due to his COPD, chronic low back pain, and hypertension. After being prepared for surgery, the patient complained of precordial chest pain. The surgery was canceled and the patient was returned to his room. Cardiac studies failed to find a reason for the chest pain which resolved later that day. What are the correct **diagnosis** codes?

Code(s): _____

1.87. This nursing home patient has extensive cellulitis of the abdominal wall. The examination performed reveals that his existing gastrostomy site is infected. He had a feeding tube inserted four months ago because of carcinoma of the middle esophagus. The physician confirmed that the responsible organism for the infection is methicillin resistant *Staph. aureus* (MRSA). What **diagnosis** codes are assigned?

Code(s): _____

# Chapter 12: Diseases of the skin and subcutaneous tissue (L00-L99)

Chapter 12 has been restructured to bring together groups of diseases that are related to one another in some way, moving from three subsections in ICD-9-CM to nine subsections in ICD-10-CM. In ICD-10-CM, these are referred to as blocks.

Instructional notes have been expanded and have several uses in this chapter. They indicate an additional code should be used to identify the organism or infectious agent. Notes also indicate that the underlying disease or associated underlying condition should be coded first. Examples are listed here:
- L14, Bullous disorders in diseases classified elsewhere, Code first underlying disease
- L97, Non-pressure chronic ulcer of lower limb, not elsewhere classified, Code first any associated underlying condition

A note under block L20-L30, Dermatitis and eczema, indicates that in this block, the terms "dermatitis" and "eczema" are used synonymously and interchangeably.

For pressure ulcers (L89), the site, laterality, and severity are specified in a single code in ICD-10-CM. The severity identified is stage 1 through stage 4. Any associated gangrene should be sequenced first.

Non-pressure chronic ulcers of lower limbs NEC (L97) are also specified by site, laterality, and severity. Code first any associated underlying condition such as:

> Any associated gangrene (I96)
> Atherosclerosis of the lower extremities (I70.23-, I70.24-, I70.33-, I70.34-, I70.43-, I70.44-, I70.53-, I70.54-, I70.63-, I70.64-, I70.73-, I70.74-)
> Chronic venous hypertension (I87.31-, I87.33-)
> Diabetic ulcers (E08.621, E08.622, E09.621, E09.622, E10.621, E10.622, E11.621, E11.622, E13.621, E13.622)
> Postphlebitic syndrome (I87.01-, I87.03-)
> Postthrombotic syndrome (I87.01-, I87.03-)
> Varicose ulcer (I83.0-, I83.2-)

## Chapter 12 Coding Cases

---

**Coding Guideline I.C.19.e. Adverse Effects, Poisoning, Underdosing and Toxic Effects**
Codes in categories T36-T65 are combination codes that include the substance that was taken as well as the intent.

No additional external cause code is required for poisonings, toxic effects, adverse effects, and underdosing codes.

---

**Coding Guideline I.C.19.e.5.a. Adverse Effect**
When coding an adverse effect of a drug that has been correctly prescribed and properly administered, assign the appropriate code for the nature of the adverse effect followed by the appropriate code for the adverse effect of the drug (T36-T50). The code for the drug should have a fifth or sixth character of 5.

---

**Coding Note:** An instructional note appears in the Tabular, under codes L27.0 and L27.1, stating to use additional code for adverse effect, if applicable, to identify drug (T36-T50 with fifth or sixth character 5).

---

**1.88.** Assign the code(s) for the following diagnosis: Dermatitis covering entire body due to antibiotics (penicillin) taken correctly as prescribed.

Code(s): _____

---

**Coding Guideline I.B.14. Documentation for BMI and Pressure Ulcer Stages**
For the body mass index (BMI) and pressure ulcer stage codes, code assignment may be based on medical record documentation from clinicians who are not the patient's provider (i.e., physician or other qualified healthcare practitioner legally accountable for establishing the patient's diagnosis), since this information is typically documented by other clinicians involved in the care of the patient (e.g., a dietitian often documents the BMI and nurses often documents the pressure ulcer stages). However, the associated diagnosis (such as overweight, obesity, or pressure ulcer) must be documented by the patient's provider. If there is conflicting medical record documentation, either from the same clinician or different clinicians, the patient's attending provider should be queried for clarification.

---

**Coding Guideline I.C.12.a.1. Pressure Ulcer Stages**
Codes from category L89, Pressure ulcer, are combination codes that identify the site of the pressure ulcer as well as the stage of the ulcer. ICD-10-CM classifies pressure ulcer stages based on severity, which is designated by stages 1-4, unspecified stage, and unstageable. Assign as many codes from category L89 as needed to identify all the pressure ulcers the patient has, if applicable.

---

**1.89.** This patient has a gangrenous pressure ulcer of the right hip with cellulitis and a pressure ulcer of the sacrum documented by the physician. The nursing assessment indicates a stage 2 pressure ulcer of the sacrum with a stage 3 decubitus ulcer of the right hip. What **diagnosis** codes are assigned?

Code(s): _____

> **Coding Guideline I.B.14 Documentation for BMI, Non-Pressure ulcers and Pressure Ulcer Stages**
> For the body mass index (BMI), depth of non-pressure chronic ulcers and pressure ulcer stage codes, code assignment may be based on medical record documentation from clinicians who are not the patient's provider, since this information is typically documented by other clinicians involved in the care of the patient (e.g., a dietitian often documents the BMI and nurses often document the pressure ulcer stages). However, the associated diagnosis (such as overweight, obesity, or pressure ulcer) must be documented by the patient's provider. If there is conflicting medical record documentation, either from the same clinician or different clinicians, the patient's attending provider should be queried for clarification.

**1.90.** Assign the code(s) for the following diagnosis: Atherosclerosis of the right ankle (native artery), with non-healing ulcer, with breakdown of the skin. The breakdown of the skin was documented only by the nurse.

Code(s): _____

**1.91.** This 35-year-old male patient presents with edema, redness, and pain of the left big toe. He did not seek treatment because he thought it would improve on its own. He does not remember any injury, but the pain has gotten progressively worse for the past week. Diagnosis: Gangrenous abscess of the entire left big toe. What **diagnosis** codes are assigned?

Code(s): _____

**1.92.** This elderly patient was seen for treatment of cellulitis in the right lower extremity. The cultures grew streptococcus B, and this was documented by the physician as the cause of the cellulitis. Patient also has stage 1 decubitus ulcer of the left buttock and stage 2 decubitus ulcer in the right gluteal region. What **diagnosis** codes are assigned?

Code(s): _____

**1.93.** The patient was seen for treatment of a fine rash that had developed on the patient's trunk and upper extremities over the last three to four days. The patient was diagnosed with hypertension seven days ago and started on Ramipril 10 mg daily. The physician determined the rash to be dermatitis due to the Ramipril. The Ramipril was discontinued and the patient was prescribed a new antihypertensive medication, Captopril. In addition, the physician prescribed a topical cream for the localized dermatitis. What **diagnosis** codes are assigned?

Code(s): _____

**1.94.** The patient was seen with extensive inflammation and irritation of the skin of both upper eyelids and under her eyebrows that was spreading to her temples and forehead. Upon questioning the patient, the physician learned that she had recently used new eye cosmetics. The physician had examined the patient during a prior visit for cystic acne. During this visit, the physician also examined the patient's cystic acne on her forehead and jawline. The patient was advised to continue using the medication previously prescribed. Diagnosis was irritant contact dermatitis due to cosmetics and cystic acne. The patient was also advised to immediately discontinue use of any make-up on the face and was given a topical medication to resolve the inflammation. What **diagnosis** codes are assigned?

Code(s): _____

**1.95.** The patient was seen for intravenous antibiotic treatment of cellulitis of the right anterior neck. The patient is also a known morphine drug abuser and exhibited considerable drug-seeking behavior and continuously requested morphine. All narcotics were discontinued and the patient exhibited no drug withdrawal symptoms.

**Diagnoses:** Cellulitis, right anterior neck; morphine drug abuse

What **diagnosis** codes are assigned?

Code(s): _____

# Chapter 13: Diseases of the musculoskeletal system and connective tissue (M00-M99)

A number of block, category, and subcategory title changes have been made in Chapter 13, for example, subsection 710-719 in ICD-9-CM, Arthropathies and Related Disorders, is called Infectious arthropathies in section M00-M25 in ICD-10-CM. Also a number of conditions have moved to this chapter from other chapters in ICD-9-CM; for example, gout moved from Chapter 3; polyarteritis nodosa moved from Chapter 7; and categories 524, Dentofacial anomalies, including malocclusion, and 526, Diseases of the jaw, moved from Chapter 9.

Bone, joint, or muscle conditions that are the result of a healed injury and recurrent bone, joint, or muscle conditions are also usually found in Chapter 13. Any current, acute injury should be coded to the appropriate injury code from Chapter 19, Injury, poisoning and certain other consequences of external causes; chronic or recurrent conditions should generally be coded with a code from Chapter 13.

The following seventh characters are required for codes in Chapter 13 that represent pathological or stress fractures in category M84.3-M84.6:

A – initial encounter for fracture
D – subsequent encounter for fracture with routine healing
G – subsequent encounter for fracture with delayed healing
K – subsequent encounter for fracture with nonunion
P – subsequent encounter for fracture with malunion
S – sequela

Seventh character A is for use as long as the patient is receiving active treatment for the fracture. Examples of active treatment are: surgical treatment, emergency department encounter, and evaluation and treatment by a new physician. Seventh character D is to be used for encounters after the patient has completed active treatment. Examples of subsequent treatment are: cast change or removal, removal of external or internal fixation device, medication adjustment, other aftercare and follow-up visits following treatment for the fracture.

As with many of the other chapters, codes have been greatly expanded to include greater anatomic specificity and laterality, and instructional notes have been expanded indicating that additional codes should be assigned for associated conditions or an underlying condition should be coded first.

Some terms have been defined in the classification. In category M66, Spontaneous rupture of synovium and tendon a spontaneous rupture is defined as one that occurs when a normal force is applied to tissues that are inferred to have less than normal strength. At category M80, Osteoporosis with current pathological fracture, a fragility fracture is defined as a fracture sustained with trauma no more than a fall from a standing height or less that occurs under circumstances that would not cause a fracture in a normal healthy bone.

## *Chapter 13 Coding Cases*

**1.96.** Assign the correct diagnosis code: Bacterial septic arthritis, right knee.

Code(s): _____

**1.97.** This young man is being treated for his ongoing juvenile rheumatoid arthritis. This condition is found only in both ankles. What **diagnosis** codes are assigned?

Code(s): _____

---

**Coding Guideline I.C.13.a. Site and Laterality**
Most of the codes within Chapter 13 have site and laterality designations. The site represents either the bone, joint, or muscle involved.

---

**Coding Note:** ICD-10-CM has three different categories for pathologic fractures: due to neoplastic disease, due to osteoporosis, and due to other specified disease.

---

**1.98.** This 76-year-old man, originally diagnosed with left upper lobe lung carcinoma 5 years ago, is seen for a fracture of the shaft of the right femur. Eight months ago, he was diagnosed with metastatic bone cancer (from the lung) and this fracture is a result of the metastatic disease. This patient's lung cancer was treated with radiation and there is no longer evidence of an existing primary malignancy. What **diagnosis** codes are assigned for this case?

Code(s): _____

---

**Coding Guideline I.C.13.d.2. Osteoporosis with Current Pathological Fracture**
Category M80, Osteoporosis with current pathological fracture, is for patients who have a current pathologic fracture at the time of an encounter. The codes under M80 identify the site of the fracture. A code from category M80, not a traumatic fracture code, should be used for any patient with known osteoporosis who suffers a fracture, even if that patient had a minor fall or trauma, if that fall or trauma would not usually break a normal, healthy bone.

---

**1.99.** Julia is an 80-year-old female with senile osteoporosis. She complains of severe back pain with no history of trauma. X-rays revealed pathological compression fractures of several lumbar vertebrae. What **diagnosis** codes are assigned?

Code(s): _____

# Chapter 14: Diseases of the genitourinary system (N00-N99)

Several block and category title changes have been made in Chapter 14; for example, subsection 617-629 in ICD-9-CM is Other Disorders of Female Genital Tract, whereas the corresponding section in ICD-10-CM, N80-N98, is Noninflammatory disorders of the female genital tract.

Codes have also moved to Chapter 14 from other chapters in ICD-9-CM; for example, ICD-9-CM code 099.40, Other nongonococcal urethritis, unspecified, moved from Chapter 1, but its ICD-10-CM counterpart, code N34.1, Nonspecific urethritis, is in Chapter 14.

Several notes are available to indicate that an additional code should be used. Some examples follow:
- N17, Acute Kidney failure – Code also associated underlying condition
- N18, Chronic kidney disease (CKD) – Code first any associated:
  - diabetic chronic kidney disease (E08.22, E09.22, E10.22, E11.22, E13.22)
  - hypertensive chronic kidney disease (I12.-, I13.-)
  - Use additional code to identify kidney transplant status, if applicable (Z94.0)
- N30, Cystitis – Use additional code to identify infectious agent (B95-B97)
- N31, Neuromuscular dysfunction of bladder, NEC – Use additional code to identify any associated urinary incontinence (N39.3-N39.4-)
- N33, Bladder disorders in diseases classified elsewhere – Code first underlying disease, such as: schistosomiasis (B65.0-B65.9)
- N40.1, Enlarged prostate with lower urinary tract symptoms (LUTS) – Use additional code for associated symptoms, when specified:
  - incomplete bladder emptying (R39.14)
  - nocturia (R35.1)
  - straining on urination (R39.16)
  - urinary frequency (R35.0)
  - urinary hesitancy (R39.11)
  - urinary incontinence (N39.4-)
  - urinary obstruction (N13.8)
  - urinary retention (R33.8)
  - urinary urgency (R39.15)
  - weak urinary stream (R39.12)

### Chapter 14 Coding Cases

**1.100.** This 40-year-old male presents with proteinuria and hematuria. Diagnosis established is chronic nephritic syndrome with diffuse membranous glomerulonephritis. What **diagnosis** code is assigned?

Code(s): _____

**1.101.** This 30-year-old female was seen with frequent urination with pain. Diagnosis: Acute suppurative cystitis, with hematuria due to E coli. What **diagnosis** codes are assigned?

Code(s): _____

**1.102.** Assign the code(s) for the following diagnosis: Premenopausal menorrhagia.

Code(s): _____

**1.103.** An 80-year-old man presented with complaints of lower abdominal pain and the inability to urinate over the past 24 hours, diagnosed as acute kidney failure due to acute tubular necrosis, caused by a urinary obstruction. The urinary obstruction was a result of the patient's benign prostatic hypertrophy. The patient was treated with medications and the acute kidney failure was resolved prior to discharge. The patient will require resection of the prostate but will return at a later date for surgery. What **diagnosis** codes are assigned?

Code(s): _____

---

**Coding Guideline I.C.14.a.2. Chronic Kidney disease and Kidney Transplant Status**
Patients who have undergone kidney transplant may still have some form of CKD, because the kidney transplant may not fully restore kidney function. Therefore, the presence of CKD alone does not constitute a transplant complication. Assign the appropriate N18 code for the patient's stage of CKD and code Z94.0, Kidney transplant status. If a transplant complication such as failure or rejection or other transplant complication is documented, see Section I.C.19.g for information on coding complications of a kidney transplant. If the documentation is unclear as to whether the patient has a complication of the transplant, query the physician.

---

**1.104.** This 45-year-old female is currently being treated for chronic kidney disease, stage 3. She has previously undergone a kidney transplant but still continues to suffer from chronic kidney disease. This patient is also treated for hypothyroidism following removal of the thyroid for thyroid carcinoma. At this time, there is no longer evidence of an existing thyroid malignancy. What **diagnosis** codes are assigned?

Code(s): _____

**1.105.** A 78-year-old female is seen with fever, malaise, and left flank pain. A urinalysis shows bacteria of more than 100,000/ml present in the urine and subsequent urine culture shows Proteus growth as the cause of the urinary tract infection. The patient was treated with intravenous antibiotics. The patient also has a history of repeated UTIs over the past several years. What **diagnosis** codes are assigned?

Code(s): _____

# Chapter 15: Pregnancy, childbirth and the puerperium (O00-O9A)

Codes have been moved from other chapters in ICD-9-CM to Chapter 15 in ICD-10-CM, for example, encounter for supervision of high-risk pregnancy has been moved from the Supplementary Classification of Factors Influencing Health Status and Contact with Health Services to ICD-10-CM Chapter 15, to category O09.

The episode of care (delivered, antepartum, postpartum) is no longer the axis of classification, but rather the trimester in which the condition occurred. Because certain obstetric conditions or complications occur during certain trimesters, not all conditions include codes for all three trimesters. And some codes do not include the trimester classification at all because the condition always occurs in a specific trimester, or the concept of trimester of pregnancy is not applicable.

The note at the beginning of the chapter defines trimesters: Trimesters are counted from the first day of the last menstrual period. They are defined as follows:
- 1st trimester - less than 14 weeks 0 days
- 2nd trimester - 14 weeks 0 days to less than 28 weeks 0 days
- 3rd trimester - 28 weeks 0 days until delivery

Chapter notes apply to the entire chapter. Note: Codes from this chapter are for use only on maternal records, never on newborn records. A code from category Z3A, Weeks of gestation, should be coded to identify the specific week of the pregnancy.

Codes from this chapter are for use for conditions related to or aggravated by the pregnancy, childbirth, or by the puerperium (maternal causes or obstetric causes).

The time frame for differentiating the abortion and fetal death codes has changed from 22 to 20 weeks (see subcategory O36.4). The time frame for differentiating early and late vomiting in pregnancy has changed from 22 to 20 weeks (see category O21). Preterm labor is defined as before 37 completed weeks of gestation (see category O60).

Certain codes in Chapter 15 require a seventh character to identify the fetus in a multiple gestation that is affected by the condition being coded. These are the applicable seventh characters:
> 0 – not applicable or unspecified
> 1 – fetus 1
> 2 – fetus 2
> 3 – fetus 3
> 4 – fetus 4
> 5 – fetus 5
> 9 – other fetus

The seventh character 0 is for single gestations and multiple gestations where the affected fetus is unspecified. Seventh characters 1 through 9 are for cases of multiple gestations to identify the fetus for which the code applies. A code from category O30, Multiple gestation must also be assigned when assigning these codes.

Multiple notes and coding guidelines apply to this chapter, so a very careful review is indicated to become proficient at coding these conditions.

One of the blocks in Chapter 21, Factors influencing health status and contact with health services is Z30-Z39, Persons encountering health services in circumstances related to reproduction. Several categories relate to the pregnant female and will be discussed in this chapter of the training. They are

| | |
|---|---|
| Z32 | Encounter for pregnancy test and childbirth and childcare instruction |
| Z33 | Pregnant state |
| Z34 | Encounter for supervision of normal pregnancy |
| Z36 | Encounter for antenatal screening of mother |
| Z3A | Weeks of gestation |
| Z37 | Outcome of delivery |
| Z39 | Encounter for maternal postpartum care and examination |

Outcome of delivery codes (Z37.0–Z37.9) are intended for use as an additional code to identify the outcome of delivery on the mother's record. It is not for use on the newborn record. These codes exclude stillbirth (P95).

### Chapter 15 Coding Cases

**Coding Note:** The note at the beginning of chapter 15 specifies the use of an additional code from category Z3A, Weeks of gestation, to identify the specific week of the pregnancy. This is found in the Alphabetic Index under Pregnancy, weeks of gestation.

**1.106.** This 36-year-old G2 P1 woman is 26-weeks pregnant and being seen for gestational hypertension. At this time, she is not having any other problems. What is the correct **diagnosis** code(s)?

Code(s): _____

**1.107.** Code the following: 16-week pregnancy with mild hyperemesis and urinary tract infection which grew out E. coli.

Code(s): _____

**1.108.** This 24-year-old woman is 3 weeks postpartum and seen today for breast pain. Final diagnosis documented as nonpurulent postpartum mastitis. What is the correct code?

Code(s): _____

---

**Coding Guideline I.C.15.a.6. Seventh Character for Fetus Identification**

Where applicable, a seventh character is to be assigned for certain categories (O31, O32, O33.3-, O33.6, O35, O36, O40, O41, O60.1, O60.2, O64, and O69) to identify the fetus for which the complication code applies.

---

**Coding Guideline I.C.15.b.5. Outcome of Delivery**

A code from category Z37, Outcome of delivery, should be included on every maternal record when a delivery has occurred. These codes are not to be used on subsequent records or on the newborn record.

---

**1.109.** This woman is G1P0 at 39 weeks with twin gestation. The delivery was complicated by nuchal cord, without compression, of fetus 2. Both infants were liveborn and healthy. What is the correct **diagnosis** code(s)?

Code(s): _____

**1.110.** This 34-year-old woman, who is G4, P3, 28 weeks, is seen today for continued follow-up of her gestational diabetes. Her diabetes has been well controlled on oral medications. What is the correct **diagnosis** code?

Code(s): _____

---

**Coding Guideline I.C.15.a.3. Final Character for Trimester**

The majority of codes in Chapter 15 have a final character indicating the trimester of pregnancy. The time frames for the trimesters are indicated at the beginning of the chapter. If trimester is not a component of a code it is because the condition always occurs in a specific trimester, or the concept of trimester of pregnancy is not applicable. Certain codes have characters for only certain trimesters because the condition does not occur in all trimesters, but it may occur in more than just one.

Assignment of the final character for trimester should be based on the provider's documentation of the trimester (or number of weeks) for the current admission/encounter. This applies to the assignment of trimester for pre-existing conditions as well as those that develop during or are due to the pregnancy. The provider's documentation of the number of weeks may be used to assign the appropriate code identifying the trimester.

Whenever delivery occurs during the current admission, and there is an "in childbirth" option for the obstetric complication being coded, the "in childbirth" code should be assigned.

---

**1.111.** Code the following **diagnosis** code(s): 20-week pregnancy with low weight gain and pre-existing essential hypertension complicating the pregnancy.

Code(s): _____

> **Coding Guideline I.C.15.n.1. Encounter for Full-term Uncomplicated Delivery**
> Code O80 should be assigned when a woman is admitted for a full-term normal delivery and delivers a single, healthy infant without any complications antepartum, during the delivery, or postpartum during the delivery episode. Code O80 is always the principal diagnosis. It is not to be used if any other code from Chapter 15 is needed to describe a current complication of the antenatal, delivery, or perinatal period. Additional codes from other chapters may be used with code O80 if they are not related to or are in any way complicating the pregnancy.

> **Coding Guideline I.C.15.n.3. Outcome of Delivery for O80**
> Z37.0, Single live birth, is the only outcome of delivery code appropriate for use with O80.

**1.112.** The patient is admitted in active labor during week 39 of pregnancy. The patient experienced no complications during her pregnancy. The patient labored for 8 hours and delivered a liveborn male over an intact perineum. Code the **diagnosis** codes only.

Code(s): _____

**1.113.** The patient, G1P0, was admitted in active labor at 38 completed weeks of gestation. The patient was dilated to 6 cm approximately 7 hours following admission. Pitocin augmentation was started and she progressed to complete dilation. A second degree perineal laceration occurred during delivery and was repaired. A female infant was delivered with Apgar scores of 9 and 9. Code the **diagnosis** codes only.

Code(s): _____

> **Coding Guideline I.C.15.f HIV. Infection in Pregnancy, Childbirth, and the Puerperium**
> During pregnancy, childbirth, or the puerperium, a patient admitted because of an HIV-related illness should receive a principal diagnosis from subcategory O98.7-, Human immunodeficiency [HIV] disease complicating pregnancy, childbirth, and the puerperium, followed by the code(s) for the HIV-related illness(es).

**1.114.** This 25-year-old patient has admitted with difficulty breathing. She has AIDS and is 21 weeks pregnant. Workup reveals Pneumocystis carinii pneumonia. What is the correct **diagnosis** code(s)?

Code(s): _____

> **Coding Guideline I.C.15.b.4. When a Delivery Occurs**
> When a delivery occurs, the principal diagnosis should correspond to the main circumstances or complication of the delivery.

> **Coding Note:** Third trimester is defined as 28 weeks 0 days until delivery.

**1.115.** The patient, G3P2, was admitted at approximately 34 weeks' gestation with a history of contractions for the last 24 hours. She was experiencing contractions every 5 to 8 minutes. An ultrasound showed an intrauterine fetal death of triplet 2 but the other two were progressing normally. The contractions stopped for approximately 24 hours and then started again. It was noted by the physician that the continued contractions were due to fetus 2. The patient was given magnesium sulfate for tocolysis which was unsuccessful. The patient also developed a fever with an infection of the amniotic sac. The patient continued to be in active labor and due to the infection was allowed to spontaneously deliver the three infants, two liveborn and one fetal death. The patient experienced no postpartum complications. Code the **diagnoses** codes only.

Code(s): _____

> **Coding Guideline I.C.15.o.1. Postpartum Period**
> The postpartum period begins immediately after delivery and continues for six weeks following delivery.

> **Coding Guideline I.C.15.o.2. Postpartum Complication**
> A postpartum complication is any complication occurring within the six-week period.

**1.116.** The patient presented three weeks after undergoing a cesarean section. The patient has a temperature of 102 degrees Fahrenheit and the cesarean section wound (operative wound) is red with minimal drainage of the incision. A wound culture grew Streptococcus group B. Discharge diagnosis: Postoperative obstetric cesarean surgical wound infection, Streptococcus, group B. Assign the correct **diagnosis** code(s). (Do not assign external cause codes.)

Code(s): _____

> **Coding Guideline I.C.15.b.4. When a Delivery Occurs**
> In cases of cesarean delivery, the selection of the principal diagnosis should be the condition established after study that was responsible for the patient's admission. If the patient was admitted with a condition that resulted in the performance of a cesarean procedure that condition should be selected as the principal diagnosis. If the reason for the admission/ encounter was unrelated to the condition resulting in the cesarean delivery, the condition related to the reason for the admission/encounter should be selected as the principal diagnosis, even if a cesarean was performed.

> **Coding Note:** ICD-10-CM provides a combination code for obstructed labor incorporating the obstructed labor with the reason for the obstruction into one code.

**1.117.** The patient, G2P1, in the 39th week of gestation was admitted with contractions occurring every 4–6 minutes. The cervix was 30% effaced with 5 cm dilation. The patient expressed her wishes for a trial vaginal delivery despite the fact that she had delivered her first child via cesarean delivery. The membranes spontaneously ruptured shortly after admission. Four hours later, the patient was given Pitocin augmentation and within 90 minutes she progressed to complete dilation and began pushing. The patient pushed for two hours and was unable to progress satisfactorily. She was taken to surgery, where a repeat low cervical cesarean section was performed for obstruction due to brow presentation. The outcome was a liveborn male infant weighing 6 pounds and 7 ounces with Apgar scores of 8 and 9. What **diagnoses** codes are coded?

Code(s): _____

> **Coding Note:** The first trimester of pregnancy is defined as less than 14 weeks 0 days.

**1.118.** The patient, G2P1, in her 12th week of pregnancy developed severe cramping and vaginal bleeding. The patient was subsequently taken to the emergency department and was admitted to the hospital. After examination, the physician documented that the patient had an incomplete early spontaneous abortion. During this pregnancy the patient had been treated for gestational hypertension of pregnancy, for which she was monitored during this hospital stay. The patient was taken to surgery where a dilation and curettage was performed. There were no complications following surgery. Code the **diagnoses** codes only.

Code(s): _____

## Chapter 16: Certain conditions originating in the perinatal period (P00-P96)

Again block and category title changes have been made in this chapter; for example, ICD-9-CM subsection 760-763 is titled "Maternal Causes of Perinatal Morbidity and Mortality," whereas the ICD-10-CM counterpart, P00-P04, is titled "Newborn affected by maternal factors and by complications of pregnancy, labor, and delivery."

While conditions originating in the perinatal period and congenital anomalies each had a specific chapter in ICD-9-CM, they are listed in a different order in ICD-10-CM. Certain conditions originating in the perinatal period is Chapter 16 and Congenital malformations, deformations, and chromosomal abnormalities is Chapter 17 in ICD-10-CM.

The phrase "fetus or newborn" used in many ICD-9-CM codes is not used in ICD-10-CM. The term "newborn" is consistently used in code titles in Chapter 16 to clarify that these codes are for use on newborn records only, never on maternal records.

The introductory notes at the beginning of the chapter provide clarification. Note: Codes from this chapter are for use on newborn records only, never on maternal records and include conditions that have their origin in the fetal or perinatal period (before birth through the first 28 days after birth) even if morbidity occurs later. Coding Guideline I.C.16.a.1 further states that Chapter 16 codes may be used throughout the life of the patient if the condition is still present. Coding Guideline i.c.16.a.4 clarifies that conditions originating in the perinatal period, and continuing throughout the life of the patient, would have perinatal codes assigned regardless of the patient's age.

A note at block P00-P04, Newborn affected by maternal factors and by complications of pregnancy, labor, and delivery also provides guidance. Note: These codes are for use when the listed maternal conditions are specified as the cause of confirmed morbidity or potential morbidity that have their origin in the perinatal period (before birth through the first 28 days after birth). Codes from these categories are also for use for newborns who are suspected of having an abnormal condition resulting from exposure from the mother or the birth process, but without signs or symptoms, and which after examination and observation, is found not to exist. These codes may be used even if treatment is begun for a suspected condition that is ruled out.

A note provides direction for coding birth weight and gestational age at categories P07 and P08 for disorders related to short gestation/low birth weight and long gestation/high birth weight. Note: When both birth weight and gestational age of the newborn are available, both should be coded with birth weight sequenced before gestational age.

Category Z38 in Chapter 21, Factors influencing health status and contact with health services classifies liveborn infants according to place of birth and type of delivery. This category is for use as the principal code on the initial record of a newborn baby. It is not to be used on the mother's record.

## *Chapter 16 Coding Cases*

> **Coding Guideline I.C.16.f. Bacterial Sepsis of Newborn**
> Category P36, Bacterial sepsis of newborn, includes congenital sepsis. If a perinate is documented as having sepsis without documentation of congenital or community acquired, the default is congenital and a code from category P36 should be assigned. If the P36 code includes the causal organism, an additional code from category B95, Streptococcus, Staphylococcus, and Enterococcus as the cause of diseases classified elsewhere, or B96, Other bacterial agents as the cause of diseases classified elsewhere, should **not** be assigned. If the P36 code does not include the causal organism, assign an additional code from category B96. If applicable, use additional codes to identify severe sepsis (R65.2-) and any associated acute organ dysfunction.

**1.119.** Assign the code(s) for the following diagnosis: 20-day-old infant was admitted with Staphylococcus aureus sepsis.

Code(s): _____

**1.120.** This full-term newborn was delivered four days ago and she was discharged with no problems. After going home she was noticed to be somewhat jaundiced, and her mother brought her to the pediatrician's office. She was diagnosed with hyperbilirubinemia and will have phototherapy provided at home. What **diagnosis** codes are assigned?

Code(s): _____

> **Coding Guideline I.C.16.a.2. Principal Diagnosis for Birth Record**
> When coding the birth episode in a newborn record, assign a code from category Z38, Liveborn infants according to place of birth and type of delivery, as the principal diagnosis. A code from category Z38 is assigned only once, to a newborn at the time of birth. If a newborn is transferred to another institution, a code from category Z38 should not be used at the receiving hospital.

**1.121.** This full-term female infant was born in this hospital by vaginal delivery. Her mother has been an alcoholic for many years and would not stop drinking during her pregnancy. The baby was born with fetal alcohol syndrome and was placed in the NICU. What **diagnosis** codes are assigned?

Code(s): _____

**Coding Guideline I.C.16.d. Prematurity and Fetal Growth Retardation**

Providers utilize different criteria in determining prematurity. A code for prematurity should not be assigned unless it is documented. Assignment of codes in categories P05, Disorders of newborn related to slow fetal growth and fetal malnutrition, and P07, Disorders of newborn related to short gestation and low birth weight, not elsewhere classified, should be based on the recorded birth weight and estimated gestational age. Codes from category P05 should not be assigned with codes from category P07.

When both birth weight and gestational age are available, two codes from category P07 should be assigned, with the code for birth weight sequenced before the code for gestational age.

A code from P05 and codes from P07.2 and P07.3 may be used to specify weeks of gestation as documented by the provider in the record.

**1.122.** Assign the codes for the following diagnosis: Premature "crack" baby born in the hospital by cesarean section to a mother dependent on cocaine. The newborn did not show signs of withdrawal. Birth weight of 1,247 g, 31 completed weeks of gestation. Dehydration. What **diagnosis** codes are assigned?

Code(s): _____

# Chapter 17: Congenital malformations, deformations and chromosomal abnormalities (Q00-Q99)

Many codes for congenital conditions and chromosomal abnormalities have been expanded in ICD-10-CM; for example, chromosomal anomalies are classified to category 758 in ICD-9-CM; however, in ICD-10-CM, there are nine categories for chromosomal abnormalities, not elsewhere classified.

Again, block, category, subcategory, and code title changes have been made in Chapter 17; for example, in ICD-9-CM, code 758.1 is titled "Patau's Syndrome," whereas the counterpart codes in ICD-10-CM are titled "Trisomy 13."

These codes are assigned when a malformation or deformation or chromosomal abnormality is documented, and the code may be the principal or first listed diagnosis on a record or a secondary diagnosis.

When no unique code is available, assign additional code(s) for any manifestations that may be present. When the code assignment specifically identifies the malformation, deformation, or chromosomal abnormality, manifestations that are an inherent component of the anomaly should not be coded separately. Additional codes should be assigned for manifestations that are not an inherent component.

Codes from Chapter 17 may be used throughout the life of the patient. If the congenital malformation or deformity has been corrected, a personal history code should be used to identify the history of the malformation or deformity. Although present at birth, malformation, deformation, or chromosomal abnormality may not be identified until later in life, and if diagnosed by the physician, it is appropriate to assign a code from codes Q00-Q99.

For the birth admission, the appropriate code from category Z38, Liveborn infants, according to place of birth and type of delivery, should be sequenced as the principal diagnosis, followed by any congenital anomaly codes, Q00-Q89.

## *Chapter 17 Coding Cases*

**1.123.** Assign the code for the following diagnosis: Frontal encephalocele with hydroencephalocele.

Code: _____

**1.124.** Assign the code(s) for the following diagnosis: Cleft palate involving both the soft and hard palate, with bilateral cleft lip.

Code(s): _____

**1.125.** Assign the code(s) for the following diagnosis: Penoscrotal hypospadias.

Code(s): _____

**1.126.** This newborn was delivered by cesarean section and transferred immediately to NICU because of previous anomalies identified via sonogram and fetal echocardiogram. The newborn male has complete transposition of the great vessels with cyanosis. The baby received IV prostaglandin and underwent uneventful corrective surgery at four days, and was discharged 10 days post surgery. What **diagnosis** codes are assigned?

Code(s): _____

# Chapter 18: Symptoms, signs and abnormal clinical and laboratory findings, not elsewhere classified (R00-R99)

Chapter 18 includes symptoms, signs, abnormal results of clinical or other investigative procedures, and ill-defined conditions regarding which no diagnosis classifiable elsewhere is recorded.

Signs and symptoms that point rather definitely to a given diagnosis have been assigned to a category in other chapters of the classification. In general, categories in this chapter include the less well-defined conditions and symptoms that, without the necessary study of the case to establish a final diagnosis, point perhaps equally to two or more diseases or to two or more systems of the body. Practically all categories in the chapter could be designated Not Otherwise Specified, Unknown Etiology, or Transient. The Alphabetic Index should be consulted to determine which symptoms and signs are to be allocated here and which to other chapters. The residual subcategories, numbered .8, are generally provided for other relevant symptoms that cannot be allocated elsewhere in the classification.

The conditions, signs, and symptoms included in Chapter 18 consist of: (a) cases for which no more specific diagnosis can be made even after all the facts bearing on the case have been investigated; (b) signs or symptoms existing at the time of the initial encounter that proved to be transient and whose causes could not be determined; (c) provisional diagnosis in a patient who failed to return for further investigation or care; (d) cases referred elsewhere for investigation or treatment before the diagnosis was made; (e) cases in which a more precise diagnosis was not available for any other reason; (f) certain symptoms, for which supplementary information is provided, that represent important problems in medical care in their own right.

### Coma Scale

Subcategory R40.2, Coma, incorporates the Glasgow coma scale (R40.21-R40.23). The coma scale codes can be used in conjunction with traumatic brain injury or sequelae of cerebrovascular disease codes. They are primarily for use by trauma registries and research use, but they may be used in any setting where this information is collected. The coma scale codes are sequenced after the diagnosis code(s). These codes, one from each subcategory (R40.21, R40.22, R40.23), are needed to complete the scale. The seventh character indicates when the scale was recorded, and it should match for all three codes:
- 0 – unspecified time
- 1 – in the field [EMT or ambulance]
- 2 – at arrival to emergency department
- 3 – at hospital admission
- 4 – 24 hours or more after hospital admission

At a minimum, report the initial score documented on presentation at the facility. This may be a score from the emergency medicine technician (EMT) or in the emergency department. If desired, a facility may choose to capture multiple coma scale scores.

Code R40.24, Glasgow coma scale, total score, should be assigned when only the total score is documented in the medical record and not the individual score(s).

## Systemic Inflammatory Response Syndrome

Systemic inflammatory response syndrome (SIRS) is classified to category R65, Symptoms and signs specifically associated with systemic inflammation and infection. Codes in this category identify SIRS of non-infectious origin with and without acute organ dysfunction and severe sepsis with and without septic shock. An instructional note indicates that the underlying condition (or underlying infection, in the case of severe sepsis) should be coded first. Sepsis is not classified to category R65. Sepsis should be coded to the infection. For example, code A41.9 should be assigned for sepsis, unspecified.

## Chapter 18 Coding Cases

**1.127.** Assign the code(s) for the following diagnosis: Right upper quadrant rebound abdominal tenderness.

Code(s): _____

---

**Coding Guideline I.C.18.e. Coma Scale**

The coma scale codes (R40.2-) can be used in conjunction with traumatic brain injury codes, acute cerebrovascular disease, or sequelae of cerebrovascular disease codes. These codes are primarily for use by trauma registries, but they may be used in any setting where this information is collected. The coma scale codes should be sequenced after the diagnosis code(s).

These codes, one from each subcategory, are needed to complete the scale. The seventh character indicates when the scale was recorded. The seventh character should match for all three codes.

At a minimum, report the initial score documented on presentation to the facility. This may be a score from the emergency medicine technician (EMT) or in the emergency department. If desired, a facility may choose to capture multiple Glasgow coma scale scores.

Assign code R40.24, Glasgow coma scale, total score, when only the total score is documented in the medical record and not the individual score(s).

---

**1.128.** Assign the Glasgow coma scale code(s) when the patient had the following documented by the EMT: Eyes do not open, no verbal response, with no motor response. The neurologist documented the following on day 2 of the hospital admission: Eyes open to sound, verbal response produced inappropriate words, and motor response with flexion withdrawal.

Code(s): _____

**1.129.** Assign the code for the following diagnosis: Microcalcification found on breast mammography.

Code(s): _____

**1.130.** Assign the code(s) for the following diagnosis: Sinoatrial bradycardia.

Code(s): _____

---

**Coding Guideline II.E. A. Symptom(s) Followed by Contrasting/Comparative Diagnoses**
When a symptom(s) is followed by contrasting/comparative diagnoses, the symptom code is sequenced first. All the contrasting/comparative diagnoses should be coded as additional diagnoses.

---

**1.131.** The patient is admitted through the emergency room with a complaint of chest pain. The EKG and laboratory tests completed in the ER are inconclusive, but an acute myocardial infarction is ruled out. During the hospital stay, the cardiovascular workup did not reveal any coronary artery disease and the patient did not want to have a cardiac catheterization study performed at this time. The patient is known to have gastroesophageal reflux disease. Given the conflicting information, the attending physician concluded the patient had "atypical chest pain due to either angina or GERD." What **diagnosis** codes are assigned?

Code(s): _____

**1.132.** The patient who has experienced a fever of 101 degrees Fahrenheit with chills was brought to the emergency room. Laboratory tests, including a complete blood count and urinalysis, were performed with normal results. The ER physician wrote the final diagnosis as "fever with chills, possible viral syndrome." What **diagnosis** code is assigned?

Code(s): _____

**1.133.** The patient is seen complaining of right upper quadrant abdominal pain. In addition, the patient is having nausea and vomited several times. Patient also has elevated blood pressure readings but a diagnosis of hypertension is not made at this visit. The patient was given an order for an outpatient sonogram. What **diagnosis** codes are assigned?

Code(s): _____

# Chapter 19: Injury, poisoning and certain other consequences of external causes (S00-T88)

In ICD-10-CM, injuries are grouped by body part rather than by categories of injury, so that all injuries of the specific site (such as head and neck) are grouped together rather than groupings of all fractures or all open wounds; for example, categories in ICD-9-CM grouped by injury such as fractures (800-829), dislocations (830-839), and sprains and strains (840-848) are grouped in ICD-10-CM by site, such as injuries to the head (S00-S09), injuries to the neck (S10-S19), and injuries to the thorax (S20-S29).

Chapter 19 encompasses two alpha characters. The **S** section provides codes for the various types of injuries related to single body regions; the **T** section covers injuries to unspecified body regions as well as poisonings and certain other consequences of external causes.

The following note refers to the entire chapter:

> Use secondary code(s) from Chapter 20, External causes of morbidity, to indicate cause of injury. Codes within the T section that include the external cause do not require an additional external cause code.

Many codes, such as fractures, include much greater specificity in ICD-10-CM. For example, some of the information that may be found in fracture codes includes the type of fracture, specific anatomical site, whether the fracture is displaced or not, laterality, routine versus delayed healing, nonunions, and malunions. Laterality and identification of type of encounter (initial, subsequent, sequela) are a significant component of the code expansion.

Seventh characters are assigned in this chapter, and are identified at the category level to indicate initial encounter, subsequent encounter, or sequela.

Fracture seventh characters are expanded to include
> A – initial encounter for closed fracture
> B – initial encounter for open fracture
> D – subsequent encounter for fracture with routine healing
> G – subsequent encounter for fracture with delayed healing
> K – subsequent encounter for fracture with nonunion
> P – subsequent encounter for fracture with malunion
> S – sequela

Some fracture categories provide for seventh characters to designate the specific type of open fracture (these designations are based on the Gustilo open fracture classification):
> B – initial encounter for open fracture type I or II (open NOS or not otherwise specified)
> C – initial encounter for open fracture type IIIA, IIIB, or IIIC
> E – subsequent encounter for open fracture type I or II with routine healing
> F – subsequent encounter for open fracture type IIIA, IIIB, or IIIC with routine healing
> H – subsequent encounter for open fracture type I or II with delayed healing
> J – subsequent encounter for open fracture type IIIA, IIIB, or IIIC with delayed healing
> M – subsequent encounter for open fracture type I or II with nonunion
> N – subsequent encounter for open fracture type IIIA, IIIB, or IIIC with nonunion

Q – subsequent encounter for open fracture type I or II with malunion
R – subsequent encounter for open fracture type IIIA, IIIB, or IIIC with malunion

In ICD-10-CM, a fracture not indicated as displaced or nondisplaced should be coded to displaced and a fracture not designated as open or closed should be coded to closed.

Seventh characters for "initial encounter" are used while the patient is receiving active treatment for the condition, for example, surgical treatment, emergency department encounter, and evaluation and treatment by a new physician.

The seventh characters for "subsequent encounter" are used for encounters after the patient has received active treatment for the condition and is receiving routine care for the condition during the healing or recovery phase, for example, cast change or removal, removal of external or internal fixation device, medication adjustment, other aftercare and follow-up visits following treatment of the injury or condition.

Seventh character S, "sequela," is for use for complications or conditions that arise as a direct result of a condition, such as scar formation after a burn. The scars are sequela of the burn. When using seventh character S, it is necessary to use both the injury code that precipitated the sequela and the code for the sequela itself. The S is added only to the injury code, not the sequela code. The seventh character S identifies the injury responsible for the sequela. The specific type of sequela (e.g., scar) is sequenced first, followed by the injury code.

The aftercare Z codes should not be used for aftercare for conditions such as injuries or poisonings, where the seventh characters are provided to identify subsequent care. For example, aftercare of an injury, assign the acute injury code with the appropriate seventh character for "subsequent encounter."

Poisoning by, adverse effects of and underdosing of drugs, medicaments and biological substances (T36-T50) includes the following note:

> *Includes:* adverse effect of correct substance properly
> administered
> > poisoning by overdose of substance
> > poisoning by wrong substance given or taken in error
> > > underdosing by (inadvertently) (deliberately) taking less
> > > substance than prescribed or instructed

Use additional code(s) for all manifestations of poisonings and assign the code for the nature of the adverse effect first followed by the code for the drug.

Use additional code for intent of underdosing:
> Failure in dosage during medical and surgical care (Y63.8-Y63.9)
> Patient's underdosing of medication regime (Z91.12-, Z91.13-)

There are combination codes for poisonings and the associated external cause (accidental, intentional self-harm, assault, undetermined), and the Table of Drugs and Chemicals groups all poisoning columns together, followed by adverse effect and underdosing. When no intent of poisoning is indicated, code to Accidental. Undetermined intent is only for use when there is specific documentation in the record that the intent of the poisoning cannot be determined.

Toxic effects of substances chiefly nonmedicinal as to source (T51-T65) provides direction to use additional code(s) for all associated manifestations of toxic effect, such as
>    Respiratory conditions due to external agents (J60-J70)

When no intent is indicated, code to Accidental. Undetermined intent is only for use when there is specific documentation in the record that the intent of the toxic effect cannot be determined.

This block has an *Excludes1* note:
>    *Excludes1*: Contact with and (suspected) exposure to toxic substances (Z77.-)

## *Chapter 19 Coding Cases*

---

**Note:** Lesson 19 will provide practice coding Chapter 19 codes. External cause codes are discussed and coded in Lesson 20 of this training. For Lesson 19, assign only diagnosis codes, not external cause codes.

---

**1.134.** The 6-month-old is seen for increased fussiness and vomiting. After significant study, the patient is diagnosed with shaken baby syndrome. What is the correct **diagnosis** code(s)? (Do not assign the external cause codes.)

Code(s): _____

---

**Coding Guideline I.C.19.a. Application of Seventh Characters in Chapter 19**
Most categories in Chapter 19 have a seventh character requirement for each applicable code. Most categories in this chapter have three seventh character values (with the exception of fractures): A, initial encounter; D, subsequent encounter; and S, sequela. Categories for traumatic fractures have additional seventh character values.

---

**Coding Guideline I.C.19.c.1. Initial vs. Subsequent Encounter for Fractures**
Traumatic fractures are coded using the appropriate seventh character for initial encounter (A, B, and C) while the patient is receiving active treatment for the fracture. Examples of active treatment are: surgical treatment, emergency department encounter, and evaluation and treatment by a new physician. The appropriate seventh character for initial encounter should also be assigned for a patient who delayed seeking treatment for the fracture or malunion.

---

**1.135.** This patient is seen for increased pain in her ankle. She has previous trimalleolar fracture of the left ankle. After evaluation she was found to have a nonunion of her left trimalleolar fracture. What is the correct **diagnosis** code(s)? (Do not assign external cause codes.)

Code(s): _____

Coding Note: ICD-10-CM categories S52, Fracture of forearm; S72, Fracture of femur; and S82, Fracture of lower leg, including ankle, have additional seventh character extensions (B, C, E, F, H, J, M, N, Q, R) to identify open fractures with the Gustilo classification. The classification is as follows:

| | |
|---|---|
| I | Low energy, wound less than 1 cm |
| II | Wound greater than 1 cm with moderate soft tissue damage |
| | High energy wound greater than 1 cm with extensive soft tissue damage |
| IIIA | Adequate soft tissue cover |
| IIIB | Inadequate soft tissue cover |
| IIIC | Associated with arterial injury |

1.136. This young man is seen today with right forearm fracture. This is found to be a displaced, compound comminuted fracture of the radial shaft. It is a type II open fracture. What is the correct **diagnosis** code? (Do not assign the external cause code.)

Code(s): _____

1.137. A 40-year-old woman is seen today to establish care. She is a complete paraplegic due to a traumatic L2 vertebral fracture five years ago. At this time, she is experiencing no problems. What is the correct **diagnosis** code(s)? (Do not assign external cause codes.)

Code(s): _____

1.138. This patient is found to have delayed healing of his traumatic mandible fracture. The fracture was at the angle of the jaw. He will be referred for additional radiologic studies. What is the correct **diagnosis** code? (Do not assign the external cause codes.)

Code(s): _____

1.139. This patient is seen emergently for a frontal skull fracture with a subsequent subdural hemorrhage. There was a 45-minute loss of consciousness at the time of the accident. What is the correct **diagnosis** code(s)? (Do not assign the external cause codes.)

Code(s): _____

1.140. Code the following diagnosis: 2 cm laceration of the left heel with foreign body. This is a current injury. (Do not assign external cause codes.)

Code(s): _____

1.141. This patient is seen in follow-up to his traumatic lateral epicondyle fracture of the right elbow. This is healing normally. What is the correct **diagnosis** code? (Do not assign external cause codes.)

Code(s): _____

**1.142.** This toddler is seen emergently for nausea and vomiting after an accidental overdose of acetaminophen. He inadvertently ate several of these when he found an open bottle at home. What is the correct **diagnosis** code(s)? (Do not assign external cause codes.)

Code(s): _____

---

**Coding Guideline I.C.19.e. Adverse Effects, Poisoning, Underdosing, and Toxic Effects**
Codes in categories T36-T65 are combination codes that include the substance that was taken as well as the intent. No additional external cause code is required for poisonings, toxic effects, adverse effects, and underdosing codes.

---

**Coding Guideline I.C.19.e.5.a. Adverse Effects**
When coding an adverse effect of a drug that has been correctly prescribed and properly administered, assign the appropriate code for the nature of the adverse effect followed by the appropriate code for the adverse effect of the drug (T36-T50). The code for the drug should have a fifth or sixth character 5. Examples of the nature of an adverse effect are tachycardia, delirium, gastrointestinal hemorrhaging, vomiting, hypokalemia, hepatitis, kidney failure, or respiratory failure.

---

**1.143.** A patient has been taking Digoxin and is experiencing nausea and vomiting and profound fatigue. The patient indicates that he has been taking the drug appropriately. The evaluation and treatment was focused on adjustment of medication only. What is the correct **diagnosis** code(s)? (Do not assign external cause codes.)

Code(s): _____

---

**Coding Guideline I.C.19.e.5.c. Underdosing**
Underdosing refers to taking less of a medication than is prescribed by a provider or a manufacturer's instruction. For underdosing, assign the code from categories T36-T50 (fifth or sixth character 6). Codes for underdosing should never be assigned as principal or first-listed codes. If a patient has a relapse or exacerbation of the medical condition for which the drug is prescribed because of the reduction in dose, the medical condition itself should be coded.

Noncompliance (Z91.12-, Z91.13-) or complication of care (Y63.8-Y63.9) codes are to be used with an underdosing code to indicate intent, if known.

---

**1.144.** This 85-year-old patient is seen in the hospital with a diagnosis of congestive heart failure due to hypertensive heart disease. Patient also has stage 5 chronic kidney failure. The patient had been prescribed Lasix previously but admits that he forgets to take his medication every day. This is due to his advanced age. What are the correct **diagnosis** codes? (Do not assign external cause codes.)

Code(s): _____

**1.145.** This 50-year-old man was in the Cardiac Cath Lab for insertion of a dual chamber pacemaker to treat his sick sinus syndrome. During the procedure the pacemaker electrode broke upon insertion. The procedure was abandoned and will be rescheduled. What is the correct **diagnosis** code(s)? (Do not assign external cause codes.)

Code(s): _____

**1.146.** This elderly woman is seen for increased right hip pain. She has a right hip prosthesis. After extensive evaluation, she is found to have an infection of the prosthesis. She will be scheduled for surgery. What is the correct **diagnosis** code? (Do not assign external cause codes.)

Code(s): _____

---

**Coding Guideline I.C.19.b.1. Superficial Injuries**
Superficial injuries such as abrasions or contusions are not coded when associated with more severe injuries of the same site.

---

**1.147.** This young snowboarder suffered a crash at a local ski area. He suffered multiple injuries and was transported to this facility for treatment. He was found to have right-sided fracture of 3 ribs, a right chest contusion and a fractured right wrist. None of his injuries required surgical intervention. What is the correct **diagnosis** code(s)? (Do not assign external cause codes.)

Code(s): _____

**1.148.** The woman is admitted for an intentional overdose of marijuana and cocaine. She sustained a fall which resulted in a left cheek and scalp laceration. After she is stabilized medically, she will be transferred to a psychiatric unit. What are the correct **diagnosis** codes? (Do not assign external cause codes.)

Code(s): _____

# Chapter 20: External causes of morbidity (V00-Y99)

This chapter permits the classification of environmental events and circumstances as the cause of injury, and other adverse effects. Where a code from this section is applicable, it is intended that it shall be used secondary to a code from another chapter of the classification indicating the nature of the condition. Most often, the condition will be classifiable to Chapter 19, Injury, poisoning and certain other consequences of external causes (S00-T88). Other conditions that may be stated to be due to external causes are classified in Chapters 1 through 18. For these conditions, codes from Chapter 20 should be used to provide additional information as to the cause of the condition.

An external cause code may be used with any code in the range of A00.0-T88.9, Z00-Z99, classification that is a health condition due to an external cause. Though they are most applicable to injuries, they are also valid for use with such things as infections or diseases due to an external source, and other health conditions, such as a heart attack that occurs during strenuous physical activity.

This chapter encompasses alpha characters V, W, X, and Y, and contains a massive expansion from ICD-9-CM. It is helpful to review the Tabular to gain an understanding of all of the possible codes available.

Assign the external cause code, with the appropriate seventh character (initial encounter, subsequent encounter, or sequela) for each encounter for which the injury or condition is being treated.

In ICD-9-CM, the late effect codes for external causes are located in various subsections of the External Cause chapter. In ICD-10-CM, all late effects of external causes are identified by the addition of the seventh character S, sequela, to the code for each intent (e.g., accident, suicide).

The transport accidents section (V00-V99) is structured in 12 groups. Those relating to land transport accidents (V01-V89) reflect the victim's mode of transport and are subdivided to identify the victim's "counterpart" or the type of event. The vehicle of which the injured person is an occupant is identified in the first two characters since it is seen as the most important factor to identify for prevention purposes. A transport accident is one in which the vehicle involved must be moving or running or in use for transport purposes at the time of the accident. The definitions of transport vehicles are provided in the classification and should be reviewed.

The following note is available with this section:
> Use additional code to identify:
>> Airbag injury (W22.1)
>> Type of street or road (Y92.4-)
>> Use of cellular telephone and other electronic equipment at the time of the transport accident (Y93.C-)

Category Y92, Place of occurrence of the external cause is for use, when relevant, to identify the place of occurrence. It is to be used in conjunction with an activity code. Place of occurrence should be recorded only at the initial encounter for treatment. Only one code from Y92 should be recorded on a medical record. Do not use place of occurrence code Y92.9 if the place is not stated or is not applicable.

Category Y93, Activity code is provided for use to indicate the activity of the person seeking healthcare for an injury or health condition, such as a heart attack while shoveling snow, which resulted from the activity or was contributed to by the activity. These codes are appropriate for use for both acute injuries, such as those from Chapter 19, and conditions that are due to the long-term, cumulative effects of an activity, such as those from Chapter 13. They are also appropriate for use with external cause codes for cause and intent if identifying the activity provides additional information on the event. These codes should be used in conjunction with codes for external cause status (Y99) and place of occurrence (Y92). The activity code is used only once, at the initial encounter for treatment. Only one code from Y93 should be recorded on the encounter.

The activity codes are not applicable to poisonings, adverse effects, misadventures, or late effects. Do not assign Y93.9, unspecified activity, if the activity is not stated.

This section contains the following broad activity categories:
Y93.0 Activities involving walking and running
Y93.1 Activities involving water and water craft
Y93.2 Activities involving ice and snow
Y93.3 Activities involving climbing, rappelling, and jumping off
Y93.4 Activities involving dancing and other rhythmic movement
Y93.5 Activities involving other sports and athletics played individually
Y93.6 Activities involving other sports and athletics played as a team or group
Y93.7 Activities involving other specified sports and athletics
Y93.A Activities involving other cardiorespiratory exercise
Y93.B Activities involving other muscle strengthening exercises
Y93.C Activities involving computer technology and electronic devices
Y93.D Activities involving arts and handcrafts
Y93.E Activities involving personal hygiene and interior property and clothing maintenance
Y93.F Activities involving caregiving
Y93.G Activities involving food preparation, cooking, and grilling
Y93.H Activities involving exterior property and land maintenance, building and construction
Y93.I Activities involving roller coasters and other types of external motion
Y93.J Activities involving playing musical instrument
Y93.K Activities involving animal care
Y93.8 Activities, other specified
Y93.9 Activity, unspecified

Category Y99, External cause status codes should be assigned whenever any other external cause code is assigned for an encounter, including an activity code, except for the events noted below. Assign a code from category Y99, External cause status, to indicate the work status of the person at the time the event occurred. The status code indicates whether the event occurred during military activity, whether a non-military person was at work, or whether an individual including a student or volunteer was involved in a non-work activity at the time of the causal event.

A code from Y99, External cause status, should be assigned, when applicable, with other external cause codes, such as transport accidents and falls. The external cause status codes are not applicable to poisonings, adverse effects, misadventures, or late effects.

Do not assign a code from category Y99 if no other external cause codes (cause, activity) are applicable for the encounter. Do not assign code Y99.9, Unspecified external cause status, if the status is not stated.

## *Chapter 20 Coding Cases*

> **Coding Note:** The seventh character must always be the seventh character in the data field. If a code that requires a seventh character is not six characters, a placeholder X must be used to fill in the empty characters.

> **Coding Guideline I.C.20.b. Place of Occurrence**
> A place of occurrence code—Y92—is used only once, at the initial encounter for treatment.

> **Coding Guideline I.C.20.c. Activity Code**
> An activity code—Y93—is used only once, at the initial encounter for treatment and should be used in conjunction with Y92, Place of occurrence.

**1.149.** Assign external cause codes for this case: An 18-year-old driver of a car collided with a pickup truck on the interstate highway. The driver confessed to using his cell phone to send a text message to his girlfriend.

Code(s): _____

**1.150.** Assign only external cause codes for this case: An Air Force officer was injured while on patrol on the military base in Afghanistan by an explosion of an IED.

Code(s): _____

**1.151.** Assign only external cause codes for this case: The patient was bitten by a dog while attempting to rescue it from an abandoned barn while performing his job at animal control.

Code(s): _____

**1.152.** Assign only external cause codes for this case: A cook in a fast food restaurant was accidently burned with hot oil while cooking French fries while on duty.

Code(s): _____

**1.153.** This 46-year-old male, working on his own home improvement projects, fell from a ladder outside of his single family home. After evaluation, it was determined that he had a non-displaced femoral neck fracture on the left side. At this time, no surgical intervention is planned. What **diagnosis** codes are assigned?

Code(s): _____

**1.154.** A patient fell from a ladder in the garage four weeks ago while working on replacing a garage door switch. The injury resulted in a fracture of L1 and L2 vertebral bodies. He is receiving physical therapy for this routine healing injury. What **diagnosis** codes are assigned?

Code(s): _____

**1.155.** A child has second- and third-degree burns of the left calf and second- and third-degree burns of the back. The patient was burned when he was running and fell into the lit fireplace in his parent's bedroom. What **diagnosis** codes are assigned?

Code(s): _____

**1.156.** This 32-year-old female was burned by hot grease in her kitchen in her condo. She is seen in the hospital's outpatient clinic for large dressing change on her left forearm. She was treated for second-degree burns to her left arm several days ago. What **diagnosis** codes are assigned?

Code(s): _____

**1.157.** This 35-year-old female patient was a driver involved in an automobile accident when she was rear-ended by another car on the interstate highway. She was seen in the emergency room complaining of pain in the arm and neck. She was brought into the hospital by the EMTs on a backboard and after proper splinting to the right arm. It was evident that there was a compound fracture present. After CT scan of the head and neck, the patient was removed from the backboard. She was treated for a displaced, compound fracture of the shaft of the right radius and ulna. She also received a collar for her cervical strain. What **diagnosis** codes are assigned?

Code(s): _____

> **Coding Guideline I.C.19.c.1. Initial vs. Subsequent Encounter for Fractures**
> Care of complications of fractures, such a malunion and nonunion, should be reported with the appropriate seventh character for subsequent care with nonunion (K, M, N) or subsequent care with malunion (P, Q, R).

**1.158.** This 10-year-old female is seen for continued pain related to her elbow fracture. Six weeks ago, this patient injured her elbow when she fell while skating at the local roller rink. After further evaluation, the attending physician found a nonunion of the previously displaced right distal humerus fracture. She will be scheduled for surgery in the next two days. What **diagnosis** codes are assigned?

Code(s): _____

> **Coding Note:** The coding note under category S61 indicates a "code also any associated wound infection" which does not provide a mandatory sequencing requirement for S61 to be sequenced ahead of the wound infection.

**1.159.** This 28-year-old female was seen for an infection due to a laceration on the palm of her right hand. Apparently, this laceration occurred five days ago. The patient reports that her hand was cut by broken glass at a restaurant, where she was a customer, drinking heavily. She is a chronic alcohol abuser and also a chronic abuser of meth. The wound will not be sutured due to the late presentation for treatment. She will, however, be placed on antibiotics to treat the infection. What **diagnosis** codes are assigned?

Code(s): _____

**1.160.** This patient is a 19-year-old college student who is brought to the emergency department by ambulance, found to be the victim of a random beating. This patient was walking in his neighborhood park when he was pulled down and then beaten during a fight. The patient was comatose when found by the paramedics but did open his eyes in response to pain; however, he has no verbal or motor response. The patient was in a coma upon admission but regained consciousness within 40 minutes of arriving in the ED, less than an hour after being found. The MRI is negative for fractures or internal bleeding. The physician describes the injury as a closed head injury with loss of consciousness of less than 1 hour. What **diagnosis** codes are assigned?

Code(s): _____

**1.161.** This is a 50-year-old female who fell down the icy front steps of her single-family house and sustained trauma to her head as well as a nondisplaced closed trimalleolar fracture of the medial and lateral malleolus of her left leg. The patient denies any loss of consciousness. Attention was directed to her head injury which, after CT scan, revealed a basilar skull fracture and a small subdural hematoma. The neurosurgeon felt that the hematoma currently did not require surgical intervention. Serial CT scans showed shrinking of the hematoma after several days. What **diagnosis** codes are assigned?

Code(s): _____

**1.162.** This patient is a 22-year-old male, admitted through the emergency department after the motorcycle he was driving (for leisure) collided with an elk on a mountain highway. The patient was wearing a helmet and suffered a minor head injury with just a short loss of consciousness reported at 15 minutes. His major injury was a displaced, cervical, C2 fracture with complete transection of the spinal cord. Upon evaluation by neurosurgery, the patient had no feeling below his shoulders, although he did admit to tingling in his arms and hands. The patient had no other apparent fractures. The patient's family was notified and arrived two days later.

Due to problems in the OR, it was necessary to transfer the patient to complete surgical stabilization. The physician's final diagnosis was stated as quadriplegia secondary to C2 vertebral fracture with spinal cord injury. What **diagnosis** codes are assigned?

Code(s): _____

# Chapter 21: Factors influencing health status and contact with health services (Z00-Z99)

Certain codes have been moved from other chapters in ICD-9-CM to Chapter 21; for example, elective, legal, or therapeutic abortions have been moved from ICD-9-CM Chapter 11, Complications of Pregnancy, Childbirth, and the Puerperium, to ICD-10-CM Chapter 21.

Several codes have been expanded in ICD-10-CM; for example, personal and family history codes have been expanded.

In addition, codes have been added for concepts that currently do not exist in ICD-9-CM; for example, category Z67 identifies the patient's blood type.

By contrast, there are also concepts that existed in ICD-9-CM that no longer exist in ICD-10-CM; for example, there is no comparable category in ICD-10-CM to ICD-9-CM category V57, Care involving use of rehabilitation procedures. For encounters for rehabilitative therapy, report the underlying condition for which therapy is being provided (such as an injury) with the appropriate seventh character indicating subsequent encounter. This change greatly impacts certain settings providing aftercare.

The note at the beginning of the chapter explains the use of the codes:

> Z codes represent reasons for encounters. A corresponding procedure code must accompany a Z code if a procedure is performed. Categories Z00-Z99 are provided for occasions when circumstances other than a disease, injury or external cause classifiable to categories A00-Y89 are recorded as "diagnoses" or "problems." This can arise in two main ways:
> a) When a person who may or may not be sick encounters the health services for some specific purpose, such as to receive limited care or service for a current condition, to donate an organ or tissue, to receive prophylactic vaccination (immunization), or to discuss a problem which is in itself not a disease or injury.
> b) When some circumstance or problem is present which influences the person's health status but is not in itself a current illness or injury.

Category Z68, Body mass index (BMI) is divided into adult and pediatric codes. The BMI adult codes are for use for persons 21 years of age or older. BMI pediatric codes are for use for persons 2–20 years of age. The percentiles listed with the codes are based on the growth charts published by the Centers for Disease Control and Prevention (CDC).

## Chapter 21 Coding Cases

**1.163.** This single newborn was born vaginally in the hospital. The baby is being treated for Rh incompatibility. The baby has type A+ blood and the mother is A-. What is the correct **diagnosis** code(s)?

Code(s): _____

**1.164.** Assign the code(s) for the following diagnosis: Medical examination of four-year-old child prior to admission to preschool.

Code(s): _____

**1.165.** Assign the code(s) for the following encounter: Patient seen for fitting of right artificial leg after patient had below-knee amputation due to medical condition.

Code(s): _____

**1.166.** Assign the code(s) for the following diagnosis: Postmenopausal osteoporosis in a 63-year-old female with a history of healed osteoporotic fracture of the ankle.

Code(s): _____

---

**Coding Guideline I.C.21.c.3. Z92.82. Status Post Administration of tPA (rtPA) in a Different Facility Within the Last 24 Hours Prior to Admission to a Current Facility**

Assign code Z92.82, Status post administration of tPA (rtPA) in a different facility within the last 24 hours prior to admission to current facility, as a secondary diagnosis when a patient is received by transfer into a facility and documentation indicates he or she was administered tissue plasminogen activator (tPA) within the last 24 hours prior to admission to the current facility. This guideline applies even if the patient is still receiving the tPA at the time he or she is received into the current facility.

The appropriate code for the condition for which the tPA was administered (such as cerebrovascular disease or myocardial infarction) should be assigned first.

Code Z92.82 is only applicable to the receiving facility record and not to the transferring facility record.

---

**1.167.** This 42-year-old male had lateral wall STEMI and was brought by ambulance to the emergency room. He received tPA and was transferred to a tertiary care center for continued care. The patient was received with the tPA infusion continuing, and immediately taken to the cardiac cath lab. What **diagnosis** codes are assigned at the receiving hospital?

Code(s): _____

**1.168.** The patient who has had his bladder removed due to carcinoma without recurrence is scheduled for a radiology procedure to evaluate the patency of his ileal conduit, including ureteropyelography using contrast media. The entire procedure is performed in the radiology suite with the radiologists' impression of "normal functioning ileal conduit." What is the correct **diagnosis** code(s)?

Code(s): _____

---

**Coding Note:** Aftercare Z codes in ICD-10-CM should not be used for aftercare of fractures. For aftercare of a fracture, assign the acute fracture code with the seventh character D (subsequent encounter).

---

**Coding Guideline I.C.20.a.2. External Cause Code Used for Length of Treatment**
Assign the external cause code, with the appropriate seventh character (initial encounter, subsequent encounter, or sequela) for each encounter for which the injury or condition is being treated.

---

**1.169.** The patient was seen in his primary care physician's office for fracture aftercare concerning the traumatic fracture of the anterior wall of the acetabulum of the right pelvis. The patient was hit by a car, knocked down, and the car ran over his pelvis. The pelvic fracture is healing appropriately. What **diagnosis** codes are assigned?

Code(s): _____

# Part II: Site-Specific Cases

## Long-Term Care Cases

Note: These cases are included for practice assigning ICD-10-CM codes. They are *not* intended to illustrate any payer specific guidelines or whether a diagnosis is reportable or not per the MDS. Further, sequencing in the following cases may not always be consistent with actual long-term care (LTC) practice. These cases are presented to practice coding, not to illustrate the correct sequencing in LTC for admissions/returns. The *Coding Clinic,* 4th Quarter, 1999 addresses LTC sequencing issues, but currently there are no comparable guidelines in ICD-10-CM.

---

**Coding Guideline I.C.21.c.3 Z79. Long-Term (Current) Drug Therapy**
Codes from this category indicate a patient's continuous use of a prescribed drug (including such things as aspirin therapy) for the long-term treatment of a condition or for prophylactic use.

---

**1.170.** This long-term multiple sclerosis patient was admitted for continuing long-term antibiotic therapy for a urinary tract infection due to E. coli. Assign the correct **diagnostic** code(s).

Code(s): _____

---

**Coding Guideline I.C.21.c.7. Aftercare**
The aftercare Z codes should not be used for aftercare for injuries. For aftercare of an injury, assign the acute injury code with the appropriate seventh character (for subsequent encounter).

---

**Coding Note:** Coding Guideline 1.C.19.a directs the coder to use D as the seventh character when coding aftercare of a condition. However, if the condition involves an open fracture, reference the Tabular List for other seventh character options using the Gustilo classification for open fractures:

        Type I – Low energy, wound less than 1 cm
        Type II – Wound greater than 1 cm with moderate soft tissue damage
        Type III – High energy wound greater than 1 cm with extensive soft tissue damage
        Type IIIA – Adequate soft tissue cover
        Type IIIB – Inadequate soft tissue cover
        Type IIIC – Associated with arterial injury

---

**1.171.** This 55-year-old male was admitted for occupational therapy (OT) following hospitalization for type I open traumatic fractures of the left radius and ulna. Assign the correct **diagnostic** code(s).

Code(s): _____

---

**Coding Note:** ICD-10-CM does not provide a separate diagnosis code for physical, occupational, and speech therapy.

---

**1.172.** A 75-year-old woman was admitted for occupational therapy (OT) following cardiac bypass surgery. She continues to have significant acute post-thoracotomy pain. Assign the correct **diagnostic** code(s).

Code(s): _____

**1.173.** This patient sustained a fractured pelvis due to a fall from his moving electric wheelchair while in the nursing facility where he resides due to multiple sclerosis. Patient is readmitted from hospital. Assign the correct **diagnostic** code(s).

Code(s): _____

---

**Coding Guideline I.C.21.c.3. Status**

A status code should not be used with a diagnosis code from one of the body system chapters, if the diagnosis code includes the information provided by the status code. For example, code Z94.1, Heart transplant status, should not be used with a code from subcategory T86.2, Complications of heart transplant. The status code does not provide additional information. The complication code indicates that the patient is a heart transplant patient.

---

**Coding Note:** Similar to the coding guideline above, when a code for adjustment or management of a device is coded, the status code does not provide additional information and should not be coded.

---

**1.174.** This patient has cardiac defibrillator in situ for ventricular fibrillation and coronary artery disease who is admitted to the nursing facility for monitoring of the defibrillator. Assign the correct **diagnostic** code(s).

Code(s): _____

**1.175.** This patient fell while walking down the hall of the nursing facility where she lives and dislocated her right wrist. This was reduced in the facility. Assign the correct **diagnostic** code(s).

Code(s): _____

**1.176.** This 48-year-old male patient was admitted for PT and OT to maintain strength for Parkinson's disease. He requires continued monitoring and is not able to live alone. He also has type 1 diabetes mellitus and COPD. Assign the correct **diagnostic** code(s).

Code(s): _____

> **Coding Guideline I.C.19.e.5. Adverse Effect**
> When coding an adverse effect of a drug that has been correctly prescribed and properly administered, assign the appropriate code for the nature of the adverse effect followed by the appropriate code for the adverse effect of the drug (T36-T50). The code for the drug should have a fifth or sixth character 5. Examples of the nature of an adverse effect are tachycardia, delirium, gastrointestinal hemorrhaging, vomiting, hypokalemia, hepatitis, renal failure, or respiratory failure.

**1.177.** A nursing home resident who is starting chemotherapy treatments at the local hospital outpatient center had adverse reaction to chemotherapy after receiving the first dose of Fluorouracil (5-FU) for carcinoma of the transverse colon. After initial stabilization at the outpatient center, the patient returned to the nursing home still requiring management of diarrhea and nausea. Assign the correct **diagnostic** code(s).

Code(s): _____

**1.178.** This patient was hospitalized for a below-the-knee amputation of the left leg. Following surgery, he developed an infection of the amputation stump which was treated during the hospitalization and the antibiotics were complete at the time of discharge. The patient is now admitted to the nursing facility for dressing changes. Assign the correct **diagnostic** code(s).

Code(s): _____

**1.179.** This 35-year-old woman is in a coma due to a late effect of ingestion of valium and alcohol. This was a suicide attempt that occurred prior to admission to the nursing facility. Assign the correct **diagnostic** code(s).

Code(s): _____

**1.180.** This patient is being treated for a pathological fracture of the right humerus due to severe senile osteoporosis. This fracture was previously diagnosed during an acute-care hospital stay. Assign the correct **diagnostic** code(s).

Code(s): _____

> **Coding Guideline I.C.19.a. Application of Seventh Characters in Chapter 19**
> Seventh character S, sequela, is used for complications or conditions that arise as a direct result of a condition such as scar formation after a burn. The scars are sequelae of the burn. When using seventh character S, it is necessary to use both the injury code that precipitated the sequela and the code for the sequela itself. The S is added only to the injury code, not the sequela code. The specific type of sequela (e.g., scar) is sequenced first, followed by the injury code.

**1.181.** This elderly gentleman has severe chronic ulcerative colitis and osteoporosis, which is due to long-term use of corticosteroid injections. Assign the correct **diagnostic** code(s).

Code(s): _____

**1.182.** Resident is admitted to the nursing home following hospitalization for acute osteomyelitis and gangrene due to a chronic nonhealing stage 3 decubitus ulcer of the right ankle. Antibiotic therapy is continued. The patient is a type 1 diabetic with peripheral vascular disease due to the diabetes. The patient also has stage 4 chronic kidney disease, hypertension, and is status post left below-the-knee amputation. PMH also includes hypercholesterolemia and chronic alcoholism which is in remission. Assign the correct **diagnostic** code(s).

Code(s): _____

**1.183.** This 81-year-old female is a resident of the nursing facility due to CHF and atrial fibrillation. She fell from the bed at the nursing facility, and was transferred to the hospital. She was readmitted to the nursing facility to resume care and to add physical therapy following open reduction and pinning of left comminuted subcapital femoral neck fracture. Assign the correct **diagnostic** code(s).

Code(s): _____

---

**Coding Guideline I.C.9.d.1. Category I69, Sequelae of Cerebrovascular Disease**
Category I69 is used to indicate conditions classified to categories I60-I67 as the causes of sequela (neurologic deficits), themselves classified elsewhere. These late effects include neurologic deficits that persist after initial onset of conditions classifiable to categories I60-I67. The neurologic deficits caused by the cerebrovascular disease may be present from the onset or may arise at any time after the onset of the conditions classifiable to categories I60-I67.

---

**Coding Note:** Coding of sequelae in ICD-10-CM generally requires two codes with the residual condition or nature of the late effect being sequenced first. An exception to this requirement is when the sequelae have been expanded to include the manifestation(s). Cerebrovascular sequelae codes have been expanded to include the manifestation and therefore require only one code for both the residual condition and the cause of the sequelae.

---

**1.184.** This nursing home resident is admitted following a hospital stay for an acute cerebral infarction. The resident will receive multiple therapies for the resulting left hemiplegia of the nondominant side, dysphasia, and facial droop. Other admitting diagnoses include GERD, rheumatoid arthritis, and early onset Alzheimer's disease with dementia and aggressive behavior. Assign the correct **diagnostic** code(s).

Code(s): _____

**1.185.** This 65-year-old female patient had been living alone and had a cerebral embolism with infarction and was admitted to the hospital. She was discharged and admitted to the nursing facility because of the residuals of altered sense of taste and left dominant hemiplegia. Assign the correct **diagnostic** code(s).

Code(s): _____

**1.186.** This 62-year-old female resident of the nursing facility has early onset Alzheimer's disease. The dementia causes her to wander off. She had a cerebral embolism with infarction while in the nursing facility, with the residuals of global aphasia and right dominant hemiplegia. She remained in the facility and was not admitted to the hospital. Assign the correct **diagnostic** code(s).

Code(s): _____

**1.187.** This 85-year-old man is admitted to the nursing facility following hospitalization for dehydration due to pneumonia. Resident is admitted for multiple therapies due to weakness because of infiltrates. He will complete the antibiotics in the nursing home for the Pseudomonas pneumonia. Resident also had progressing dementia resulting from Parkinson's disease and he realized that it was getting more difficult to remain in his own home and agreed to admission. His past medical history includes mitral valve regurgitation, kyphosis, mild asthma, and type 2 diabetes. Assign the correct **diagnostic** code(s).

Code(s): _____

**1.188.** This patient is admitted to the nursing facility for PT and OT following hospitalization for an infected hip prosthesis that was performed two months prior. Resident was found to have vancomycin resistant enterococcus (VRE) that will require antibiotic therapy for six weeks via PICC line. The hospital discharge summary also included the following diagnoses: BPH with urinary obstruction, situational depression with agitation, hypertension, atrial fibrillation treated with Coumadin with INRs monthly. Assign the correct **diagnostic** code(s).

Code(s): _____

---

**Coding Guideline I.C.4.a.3. Diabetes Mellitus and the Use of Insulin**
If the documentation in a medical record does not indicate the type of diabetes but does indicate that the patient uses insulin, code E11, Type 2 diabetes mellitus, should be assigned. Code Z79.4, Long-term (current) use of insulin, should also be assigned to indicate that the patient uses insulin. Code Z79.4 should not be assigned if insulin is given temporarily to bring a type 2 patient's blood sugar under control during an encounter.

---

**1.189.** A resident was admitted to the nursing facility following foot amputation due to diabetic peripheral vascular disease. PT and OT were ordered with the plan for the resident to return home. Staff is to change dressings and report any suture site breakdown to the physician. Other diagnoses include gastroparesis due to type 2 diabetes (receiving insulin), mitral valve regurgitation with aortic stenosis, inguinal hernia, generalized DJD and COPD. Assign the correct **diagnostic** code(s).

Code(s): _____

## *Home Healthcare Cases*

Note: These cases are included for practice assigning ICD-10-CM codes. They are *not* intended to illustrate any payer specific guidelines or whether a diagnosis is reportable or not per OASIS.

---

**Coding Note:** Superficial injuries, such as abrasions or contusions are not coded when associated with more severe injuries of the same site.

---

**1.190.** This 75-year-old woman is receiving continuing care for multiple facial lacerations, abrasions, and contusions. She was previously treated in the hospital's emergency department for these injuries. Assign the correct **diagnostic** code(s).

Code(s): _____

**1.191.** This 88-year-old gentleman is receiving home care for his coronary artery disease and the cardiac pacemaker placed during his hospitalization last week. He continues to gain strength but requires wound checks, dressing changes, and medication management ongoing. Assign the correct **diagnostic** code(s).

Code(s): _____

---

**Coding Guideline I.C.2.k. Malignant Neoplasm Without Specification of Site**
Code C80.1, Malignant (primary) neoplasm, unspecified, equates to Cancer, unspecified.
This code should only be used when no determination can be made as to the primary site of a malignancy. This code should be rarely used in the inpatient setting.

---

**1.192.** This woman is being treated for a severe allergic reaction to chemotherapy due to cancer. The specific drug is Fluorouracil. Assign the correct **diagnostic** code(s).

Code(s): _____

**1.193.** This patient is admitted to home care for physical therapy three times a week and for surgical dressing changes two times a week after falling from an escalator at the mall. The patient is status-post traumatic right subtrochanteric hip fracture and is receiving continued care for this fracture with routine healing. Assign the correct **diagnostic** code(s).

Code(s): _____

**1.194.** This patient is a 65-year-old female admitted to home care following a hip replacement for osteoarthritis of the left hip. Patient was placed on Coumadin following surgery and has a refill for the Coumadin to continue several weeks postoperatively. Nurses are to do PT/PTT to monitor Coumadin levels, to change dressings, to watch for healing and signs of infection, and to report to the physician weekly. PT is providing gait training for walking difficulties. Assign the correct **diagnostic** code(s).

Code(s): _____

**1.195.** Home care skilled nursing visits are ordered for a patient who is on home oxygen for chronic obstructive pulmonary disease. Assign the correct **diagnostic** code(s).

Code(s): _____

**1.196.** This patient is admitted to home care with cellulitis of the right arm and is receiving IV antibiotics via a PICC line with routine PICC line maintenance. Assign the correct **diagnostic** code(s).

Code(s): _____

**1.197.** This female patient is admitted to home care following modified radical mastectomy for adenocarcinoma of the lower-outer quadrant of the right breast. Nursing services were ordered and provided for wound healing and dressing changes. Patient will be receiving chemotherapy in the following weeks. Assign the correct **diagnostic** code(s).

Code(s): _____

**1.198.** Patient is a 67-year-old woman, admitted to home care for physical therapy only for gait abnormality, following a total knee replacement of her right knee for osteoarthritis of the same knee. Patient had osteoarthritis of that particular joint only. Assign the correct **diagnostic** code(s).

Code(s): _____

**1.199.** An 80-year-old woman is admitted to home care following a hip replacement after traumatic closed fracture of the left hip, after she slipped on the ice in front of the grocery store. Since returning home the patient has developed a superficial wound infection at the incision site which will be addressed by home care staff. The physician has ordered wound care three times per week and gait training two times per week for her gait abnormality. Assign the correct **diagnostic** code(s).

Code(s): _____

**1.200.** Home healthcare nurses have been ordered to do monthly Foley catheter changes on this 70-year-old patient with a long-standing neurogenic bladder. Nurses are providing only Foley catheter changes. Assign the correct **diagnostic** code(s).

Code(s): _____

**1.201.** Home healthcare has been ordered by the patient's physician for this 75-year-old male who has had a cholecystectomy for acute cholecystitis. He had a drain placed at surgery to drain intra-abdominal fluid. Nurses are to monitor the drain output, watch for signs of infection, and provide dressing changes and remove drain per order. Assign the correct **diagnostic** code(s).

Code(s): _____

**1.202.** Patient is admitted to home care following a hospitalization for congestive heart failure, peripheral vascular insufficiency, and hypothyroidism. Skilled nursing is ordered for observation, weights, and medication management. Assign the correct **diagnostic** code(s).

Code(s): _____

**1.203.** Patient is discharged from the hospital after a problem with type 1 diabetes in ketoacidosis. Currently the diabetes is poorly controlled. Patient has a new insulin pump and is struggling to maintain glucose control. Skilled nursing is to both monitor glucose levels and provide dietary counseling and insulin pump training. Assign the correct **diagnostic** code(s).

Code(s): _____

**1.204.** Patient is admitted to home care following CABG for coronary artery disease. Nursing is following to provide skilled observation of cardiac status and wound care. Assign the correct **diagnostic** code(s).

Code(s): _____

**1.205.** An 80-year-old female is discharged from the hospital following surgical treatment for a malignant neoplasm of the sigmoid colon. The physician indicates that the patient will be undergoing chemotherapy for sigmoid cancer. Skilled nursing services are ordered for this patient three times a week for six weeks to teach colostomy care and assess the patient's compliance with medications. Assign the correct **diagnostic** code(s).

Code(s): _____

Part II

> **Coding Guideline I.C.19.a. Application of Seventh Characters in Chapter 19**
> The aftercare Z codes should not be used for aftercare of conditions such as injuries or poisonings, where seventh characters are provided to identify subsequent care. For example, for aftercare of an injury, assign the acute injury code with the seventh character D (subsequent encounter).

> **Coding Guideline I.C.19.c. Coding of Traumatic Fractures**
> A fracture not indicated as open or closed should be coded to closed. A fracture not indicated whether displaced or not displaced should be coded to displaced.

**1.206.** An 85-year-old independent female fell in her home, sustaining a left hip fracture. An open reduction with internal fixation was performed seven days ago. The patient was discharged home where her sister now cares for her. The patient is non-weight bearing on left lower extremity but can perform supervised pivot transfers with contact guard assist in and out of bed. The physician orders the agency to provide physical therapy for gait training because of gait abnormality, and exercise three times per week for four weeks. Assign the correct **diagnostic** code(s).

Code(s): _____

**1.207.** An 83-year-old female is admitted by the HHA following discharge from the hospital. The patient is seven days status post left total hip replacement due to generalized osteoarthritis. She developed a mildly exudated postop wound infection (MRSA), with partial separation of her surgical incision with external wound dehiscence. She was discharged from the hospital with IV antibiotics. This is the patient's initial episode of home healthcare.

**Skilled Nursing Need:** The patient's physician ordered daily skilled nursing visits for three weeks to treat her infected left hip surgical wound. The specific skilled nursing services ordered by the physician include the following:
- Monitor the wound for increasing signs and symptoms of infection;
- Administer IV antibiotics daily for 21 days; and
- Teach the patient's daughter to perform IV administration and wound care.

**Therapy Need:** The patient's physician ordered physical therapy services for gait training and strengthening exercises two times a week for four weeks. Ambulation is limited due to non-weight bearing status of her left lower extremity. The patient can perform supervised pivot transfers with contact guard assistance in and out of bed. Her daughter will be staying with her until her mobility improves. Assign the correct **diagnostic** code(s).

Code(s): _____

**1.208.** A 66-year-old left-handed woman who lives alone is discharged from the hospital three days after a right, modified radical mastectomy for breast cancer. She has residual weakness of her left arm, due to H/O stroke and is unable to care for her breast wound. Her medications include Tamoxifen for breast cancer chemotherapy and pain medications. Her physician reports that the patient's breast cancer is not resolved and the surgical drain is scheduled to be removed in several days.

**Skilled Nursing Need:** The patient's physician ordered skilled nursing visits daily for 10 days until the surgical drain is removed, then three times a week for four weeks to provide surgical wound care and supervision of the exercises ordered to improve her right shoulder range of motion and to monitor for any signs of infection.

**Skilled Therapy Need:** Skilled therapy services are not required or ordered by the patient's physician. The nurse will supervise the patient's performance of the exercises ordered to improve her shoulder range of motion on the affected side. Assign the correct **diagnostic** code(s).

Code(s): _____

**1.209.** A 70-year-old male is admitted to home health following discharge from an acute rehab facility. The patient received two weeks of physical therapy following his hospitalization for an acute CVA with infarct. Although his functional ability is improved, he is unable to ambulate due to monoparesis of his right lower leg, which is affecting his dominant right side. He has the ability to wheel independently in his wheel-chair. The patient requires physical therapy to regain his normal gait. His physician orders seven weeks of home health skilled therapy due to Monoplegia of lower limb affecting his dominant side.

**Skilled Nursing:** The HHA did not receive an order from the patient's physician to provide skilled nursing services. The patient's initial comprehensive assessment visit by the HHA did *not* identify a skilled nursing need.

**Therapy Need:** The patient's physician ordered physical therapy for gait evaluation/ training and strengthening exercises three times per week for four weeks, then two times per week for three weeks. The patient is currently wheelchair dependent (chairfast). He is unable to ambulate but he is able to wheel independently in his wheel-chair. This is his first episode of home healthcare. Twenty therapy visits are ordered by his physician for this episode of care. Assign the correct **diagnostic** code(s).

Code(s): _____

## *Hospital Inpatient Cases*

---

**Coding Guideline I.C.1.d.1.a. Sepsis**
For a diagnosis of sepsis, assign the appropriate code for the underlying systemic infection. If the type of infection or causal organism is not further specified, assign code A41.9, Sepsis, unspecified organism.

A code from subcategory R65.2, Severe sepsis, should not be assigned unless severe sepsis or an associated acute organ dysfunction is documented.

---

**1.210.** The following documentation is from the health record of a 71-year-old male patient.
**Discharge Summary**
**History and Physical Findings:** This 71-year-old male is a nursing home resident as a result of a cerebrovascular accident two years ago. He has had numerous hospital admissions for pneumonia and other infectious complications. On the day of admission, the patient was noted to be clammy, with tachypnea, to have decreased level of responsiveness, and to show increased fever. He was seen in the ER, where evaluation revealed the presence of probable urinary tract infection and sepsis. The patient was also found to have renal insufficiency with BUN and creatinine elevated. His WBC count was 23,000 with decreased hemoglobin and hematocrit. He was admitted for treatment of E. coli sepsis. Physical examination revealed an elderly male who was aphasic and had right-sided hemiplegia (he is right-handed), both from a previous CVA. The heart had a regular rhythm. The lungs were clear. The abdomen was soft.

**Significant Lab, X-ray, and Consult Findings:** Follow-up chemistry showed progressive decline in the BUN and creatinine to near normal levels. Initial white blood cell count was 23,700. Final blood count was 9,000. The urinalysis showed too numerous to count white cells. The urine culture had greater than 100,000 colonies of E. coli and Group B strep, which revealed the cause of the UTI. Repeated blood cultures grew E. coli with the same sensitivities as that of the urine. There were no acute abnormalities noted. EKG showed sinus tachycardia and low lead voltage, otherwise was normal and unchanged.

**Course in Hospital:** The patient was initially started empirically on Primaxin. He underwent fluid rehydration and his electrolytes were followed closely. Electrolytes improved through his hospital stay. He was continued on IV Primaxin until the date of discharge, when he was changed to Cipro by tube. All of the bacteria grown in the urine and in the blood were sensitive to the Cipro. The chest x-ray showed no change from previous admissions, and he was followed closely with additional oxygen as needed. The patient does have a history of chronic obstructive lung disease and has required intermittent oxygen therapy at the nursing home. At this time, the patient had reached maximal hospital benefit. He was switched to oral antibiotics. He was to continue on tube feedings, which he was tolerating quite well. The patient was discharged back to the nursing home on 5/4. Assign the correct **diagnostic** code(s).

**Discharge Diagnoses:**
1. E. coli sepsis
2. UTI, due to E. coli, and Group B strep
3. Renal insufficiency
4. Chronic obstructive lung disease
5. CVA with right hemiplegia

Code(s): _____

---

**Coding Guideline I.C.2.c.2. Anemia Associated with Chemotherapy, Immunotherapy and Radiation Therapy**

When the admission/encounter is for management of an anemia associated with an adverse effect of the administration of chemotherapy or immunotherapy and the only treatment is for the anemia, the anemia code is sequenced first, followed by the appropriate codes for the neoplasm and the adverse effect (T45.1x5), Adverse effect of antineoplastic and immunosuppressive drugs).

When the admission/encounter is for management of an anemia associated with an adverse effect of radiotherapy, the anemia code should be sequenced first, followed by the appropriate neoplasm code and code Y84.2, Radiological procedure and radiotherapy as the cause of abnormal reaction of the patient, or of later complication, without mention of misadventure at the time of the procedure.

---

**1.211.** A patient with known carcinoma of the pancreatic head is admitted with an Hgb of 9.1. She has been receiving Docetaxel chemotherapy and the physician diagnoses this new anemia as an adverse effect of the chemotherapy. The patient is treated with darbepoetin alpha and IV iron. The patient is discharged with an improvement in the Hgb to 11.3. Assign the correct **diagnostic** code(s).

Code(s): _____

**1.212.** The following documentation is from the health record of an 85-year-old female patient.

**Discharge Summary:** This 85-year-old female patient was noted to have three to four falls in the past two months at ABC Nursing Home. Patient fell yesterday from her parked wheelchair and hit the left frontal temporal area of her head causing a contusion. For this reason, the patient was brought to the hospital for observation and further workup. The patient's exam was remarkable for moderate ataxia. Past medical history includes senile dementia – Alzheimer's, late onset type, depression and emphysema. Current medications include Zoloft and Theophylline. CT scan of the brain noted that the patient had multiple masses in the brain due to metastatic disease. It was felt that the patient's ataxia was most likely due to the metastatic disease of the brain. These results were discussed with the patient's family. After much discussion regarding the treatment options, the family decided that they did not want the patient to undergo further tests and/or evaluation. It was the family's decision that the patient be transferred back to the nursing home and put under hospice care. Assign the correct diagnostic code(s).

Code(s): _____

**1.213.** The following documentation is from the health record of a 58-year-old male patient.
**Discharge Diagnoses:**
1. Carcinoma of the lung, right upper lobe, currently undergoing chemotherapy
2. Type 2 diabetes, with neuropathy and nephropathy
3. Hyperlipidemia
4. Hepatomegaly

**History:** This patient is a 58-year-old male who presented for outpatient chemotherapy. He had surgery for lung cancer three months ago and is now undergoing chemotherapy with Taxol and carboplatin, including dexamethasone as part of his chemotherapy and prophylaxis for nausea. He has done very well with the outpatient chemotherapy. When he presented for treatment on the day of admission, he was found to be hypoglycemic. He is a known type 2 diabetic which is also complicated by neuropathy and nephropathy. Due to his blood glucose levels, it was decided to postpone this chemotherapy session and he was admitted for control of his diabetes. Dr. Johnson consulted with the patient to manage his diabetes regimen. He has been on 70/30 insulin, 25 units in the morning and 15 units in the evening for several years. An IV insulin drip was started and he also had q 1 hour Accu-Checks. His hepatomegaly has enlarged from the last time that I saw him. Question whether this is fatty infiltration due to poor diabetes control, or whether there is now some involvement with metastatic carcinoma.

**Lab Data:** Sodium 128, potassium 5.5, chloride 89, BUN 13, creatinine 0.8, glucose range 30-460, with final glucose of 210. Calcium 9.4, WBC 9.8, hemoglobin 11.6, hematocrit 34.3, platelets 277,000.

**Plan:** One difficulty here is the cyclic nature of his chemotherapy treatment regimen, likely to produce major shifts in his glucose, which is already difficult to control. The patient will need to monitor his glucose levels closely. He is discharged on 70/30 insulin, 35 units in the morning and 20 units in the evening. He is to follow up with me for further chemotherapy in the oncology clinic next week. Assign the correct **diagnostic** code(s).

Code(s): _____

**1.214.** The following documentation is from the health record of an 87-year-old female patient.

**Discharge Summary**

**History of Present Illness:** The patient is an 87-year-old female who was admitted from a nursing home with congestive heart failure, dehydration as well as urinary tract infection and thrombocytopenia with petechial hemorrhage. On admission she was found to have a platelet count of 77,000 and a Hematology consult was done. The patient denied any bleeding diathesis in the past. She stated that she had recent bruising of the hands related to needle sticks, but otherwise has not had any past history of any bleeding disorder. No specific history of hematuria, hematemesis, gross rectal bleeding, or black stools.

**Past Medical History:** Significant for congestive heart failure, diabetes

**Medications:** Coreg, isosorbide, Actos, digoxin, glyburide, hydralazine, furosemide, Ditropan, and potassium

**Family History:** No family history of any bleeding disorder

**Physical Examination:** She is an elderly-appearing white female, somewhat short of breath, using supplemental oxygen. Examination of the head and neck revealed no scleral icterus. Throat was clear. Tongue was papillated. There was no thyromegaly or JVD. There was no cervical supraclavicular, axillary, or inguinal adenopathy. Chest examination revealed rales, bilaterally. There were decreased breath sounds at the right base. There were coarse rales heard in the right midlung field. Heart exam showed rhythm was irregular. Abdomen exam was difficult to perform. I was unable to palpate the liver or spleen. Bowel sounds were active. Extremities revealed no clubbing, cyanosis, or edema. There were diffuse ecchymoses, especially in the dorsum of the right hand.

**Laboratory Studies:** Hematocrit was 43, white count 9,000 with 82% neutrophils, and the platelet count 77,000. The MCCV was 102. Creatinine was 1.7. Bilirubin was 1.7. The alkaline phosphatase was 122. AST 498, ALT 493, and albumin 3.6. The prothrombin time was 18 seconds, the PTT was 25 seconds. The chest x-ray showed a right pleural effusion.

**Course in Hospital:** The patient was admitted and started on IV fluids. Her diuretics were increased, and she showed a good response and better control of her congestive heart failure. Hematology consult recommended holding platelet transfusion unless there was evidence of active bleeding. No platelets were given during this admission.

The patient was discharged back to the nursing home on day six in improved condition to continue with the same medication regimen as previous to hospitalization. Assign the correct **diagnostic** code(s).

**Final Diagnoses:**
1. Congestive heart failure
2. Dehydration
3. Primary thrombocytopenia with petechial hemorrhage and hematoma of the eyelids and bilateral arms and hands
4. Urinary tract infection
5. Type 2 diabetes mellitus

Code(s): _____

> **Coding Guideline I.C.9.a.1. Hypertension with Heart Disease**
> Heart conditions classified to I50.- or I51.4-I51.9 are assigned to a code from category I11, Hypertensive heart disease, when a causal relationship is stated (due to hypertension) or implied (hypertensive). Use an additional code from category I50, Heart failure, to identify the type of heart failure in those patients with heart failure.

**1.215.** The following documentation is from the health record of an 85-year-old female patient.

### Discharge Summary

**Admit Date:** 12/10/XX
**Discharge Date:** 12/22/XX

**Discharge Diagnoses:**
1. Hypertensive left heart failure with acute pulmonary edema
2. Myocardial infarction ruled out
3. Chronic obstructive pulmonary disease
4. Pseudomonas pneumonia

**History of Present Illness:** This 85-year-old female was admitted via the Emergency Room from the nursing home with shortness of breath, confusion, and congestion. There was no history of fever or cough noted. Patient also has a history of COPD. Prior to admission, the patient was on the following medications: Prednisone, Lasix, Benicar, and Colace. Patient had a long history of tobacco dependence prior to admission to the nursing home.

**Physical Examination:** Blood pressure 140/70, heart rate of 125 per minute, respirations were 30, temperature of 101.4. The eyes showed postsurgical eyes, nonreactive to light. The lungs showed bilaterally bibasilar crackles. The heart showed S1 and S2, with no S3. The abdomen was soft and nontender. The extremities showed leg edema. The neurological exam revealed no deficits and she was alert ×3.

**Hospital Course:** Basically, this patient was admitted to the coronary care unit with acute pulmonary edema, rule out myocardial infarction. Serial cardiac enzymes were done, which were within normal limits, therefore ruling out myocardial infarction. A chest x-ray performed on the day before admission confirmed left heart failure and pneumonia.

The patient was started on Unasyn and Tobramycin for the pneumonia, which improved. The left heart failure, however, was not improving with administration of Lasix. The patient was not taking foods and liquids well, and, at the family's request, she was made DNR. On hospital day 12, she was found without respirations, with no heart sounds, and pupils were fixed. She was declared dead by the physician, and the family was notified. Assign the correct **diagnostic** code(s).

Code(s): _____

**1.216.** The following documentation is from the health record of a 69-year-old female.

**History of Present Illness:** The patient is a 69-year-old female with previous MI, known hypertensive, who started complaining of cough, chills, and fever about 4 days prior to admission. One day prior to admission, she started to complain of progressive dyspnea. She went to the ER and was noted to be extremely dyspneic and wheezing. She was given an aerosol treatment with good response. However, chest x-ray showed evidence of bilateral lower pneumonia with a PO2 of 66 and white blood cell count of 12,400. The patient was subsequently admitted. The patient has been taking Methyldopa 500 mg. bid, Ascriptin 1 tablet daily, Transderm Nitro 5 once daily, Capoten 30 mg. bid, and Lanoxin 0.725 mg. daily. The patient had an inferior wall myocardial infarction three years ago and chronic, mild congestive heart failure. She is known to have chronic anxiety problems and has been under the care of the Mental Hygiene Clinic.

**Physical Examination:** Revealed a well-developed, well-nourished female whose respirations had improved since the aerosol therapy was given. Blood pressure is somewhat elevated. Respirations 24. Pulse 110/minute. HEENT: Unremarkable. No carotid bruits. No distended neck veins. Chest: No deformity. Equal expansion. Lungs: Crepitant rales over the lower half of hemithorax. No wheezing. No pericardial or pleural rub noted. Heart: Regular rhythm. No murmurs. Abdomen: Soft. Liver, spleen and kidneys not enlarged. No tenderness. Extremities: No clubbing. No cyanosis. Peripheral pulses strong and equal.

**Impression:** Lobar pneumonia. Previous inferior wall myocardial infarction. Hypertension. Chronic anxiety.

**Hospital Course:** Sputum smear showed moderate white blood cells, many epithelial cells and many mixed respiratory microflora. Sputum culture showed normal growth. Blood cultures after 10 days showed no growth. Chest x-ray report revealed acute congestive cardiac failure. Significant improvements in congestive heart failure noted on second x-ray, but not complete resolution, although the pneumonia has resolved. EKG showed right bundle branch block with old inferior myocardial infarction. This patient's previous medications were continued during hospitalization.

After cultures were obtained, she was empirically started on IV Kefzol and aerosolized bronchodilator therapy consisting of Alupent. She remained afebrile during her stay in the hospital. She had no further wheezing after 24 hours, but continued to have mild crepitant rales in both bases. She had one episode of mild angina pains relieved by nitroglycerin during her stay. With improvement in her respirations and x-ray findings, she was discharged. Her BP was 154/110 on discharge, but this is not considered unusual since her BP is quite unstable as an outpatient, with variable high and low readings. This will, however, be followed up in the office. Assign the correct **diagnostic** code(s).

**Final Diagnoses:**
1. Bilateral pneumonia
2. Old myocardial infarction with angina
3. Hypertension
4. Chronic anxiety
5. Acute on chronic diastolic congestive heart failure

Code(s): _____

**1.217.** The following documentation is from the health record of a 33-year-old female patient.

**OB Record**
**Admit Note 2/27**
This is a 33-year-old G2 P0, with an estimated delivery date of 2/28, and estimated gestational age of 40 weeks. She presents for induction secondary to gestational diabetes mellitus. The diabetes has been managed by diet throughout the pregnancy. The patient also has diastasis recti that occurred three weeks ago, which has kept her at bedrest since that time. PNL: O positive, rubella immune. PE: AVSS, Abdomen FH 40 cm, EFW 3800-4000 grams. Cervix is closed/50%/-3/post/ceph. Plan is for Pitocin induction with epidural at the beginning of active labor.

**Progress Note 2/28 09:15**
Patient is having uterine contractions every 3-8 minutes. Cervix is 1 cm/100%/floating. Patient desires not to start Pitocin yet. Feels that she is in labor. FHR reactive, baseline 120's with accelerations.

**Progress Note 2/28 19:25**
Patient's uterine contractions have resolved. Cervix unchanged. Discussed options, would like to go home to sleep and return in a.m. for Pitocin induction. Discharged home for tonight to sleep. Admit in a.m., start IV Pitocin as per protocol and clear liquid diet. Assign the correct **diagnostic** code(s).

Code(s): _____

**1.218.** The following documentation is from the health record of an 18-day-old baby boy.

**Discharge Summary**
This is an 18-day-old male infant, who was admitted after he was noticed to be developing omphalitis. He was immediately placed on intravenous Cefotaxime and Ampicillin, later changed to Cefotaxime and Clindamycin. A culture taken from the umbilical stump grew Staphylococcus aureus (MRSA) and Group H Streptococcus.

After the first day, there was great improvement and the patient continued to improve completely. Now there is no redness or swelling whatsoever. The child has remained afebrile, has continued to eat very well. He shows no sign of abdominal tenderness or peritonitis. I feel that we have treated this well. He has had five days of intravenous antibiotics. I will finish the treatment with Keflex by mouth seeing that both Streptococcus pyogenes and Staphylococcus aureus are sensitive. The mother will watch the child closely and let me know if any problems occur. I have instructed her to watch for any more redevelopment of the redness, swelling, or discharge. We will recheck this in two weeks for one-month checkup. Assign the correct **diagnostic** code(s).

Code(s): _____

---

**Coding Guideline I.C.19.e. Adverse Effects, Poisoning, Underdosing, and Toxic Effects**
Codes in categories T36–T65 are combination codes that include the substance that was taken as well as the intent. No additional external cause code is required for poisonings, toxic effects, adverse effects, and underdosing codes.

When coding a poisoning or reaction to the improper use of a medication (e.g., overdose, wrong substance given or taken in error, wrong route of administration), first assign the appropriate code from categories T36–T50. The poisoning codes have an associated intent as their fifth or sixth character (accidental, intentional self-harm, assault, and undetermined). Use additional code(s) for all manifestations of poisonings.

---

**1.219.** The following documentation is from the health record of a 17-year-old male patient.

**History of Present Illness:** The patient is a 17-year-old white male who was brought to the ED after being found in the town park. The patient was in restraints and accompanied by two police officers. The patient was combative and aggressive, threatening physical harm to himself as well as the physician and hospital staff. The patient has a long history of alcohol and drug abuse, was in the local treatment center, and walked off campus two days ago.

**Allergies:** NKDA

**PMH:** Attention deficit hyperactivity disorder (ADHD), amphetamine drug and alcohol dependence, unsocialized aggressive behavior

**Family History:** Noncontributory

**ROS:** As above

**Physical Examination:** Vital signs: temp. 100.1 degrees, BP 144/88 mmHg; General: alternating between lethargy and combativeness; HEENT: pupils pinpoint, 1 mm bilaterally; Skin: cool, clammy to touch, feet and hands cold, slightly diaphoretic; Heart: rate tachy, no murmurs; Lungs: clear, respiratory rate 28 and shallow; Abdomen: benign; Neurological: mental status as above; follows commands inconsistently, responds to voice; cranial nerves: pupils as noted, gag intact; motor: moving all four extremities with equal power; sensory: responds to touch in all four extremities; deep tendon reflexes +3 throughout, but plantar reflexes down going bilaterally.

**Laboratory:** U/A shows 2+ blood, done after Foley catheter was placed; drug screen + for amphetamines; ETOH 45 mg/100 ml; ABG within normal limits; EKG sinus tachycardia.

**Hospital Course:** Family was contacted, IV fluids were initiated for dehydration and tachycardia, and the patient was admitted to ICU with suicide protocol, Ativan 1–2 mg IV q 2 hours prn. He was maintained on soft restraints with checks every 15 minutes and monitored with telemetry and neuro checks through the night. By the morning he was no longer tachycardic. By hospital day three he was medically stable, but still saying he wants to "kill himself." Psychiatric consult requested.

**Disposition:** Discharge to psych. Psychiatric liaison service agreed to accept him in transfer to the inpatient adolescent psychiatric unit at children's hospital. Assign the correct **diagnostic** code(s).

**Discharge Diagnoses:**
1. Drug overdose with amphetamines and alcohol
2. Suicide attempt
3. Alcohol intoxication

Code(s): _____

**1.220.** The patient is being seen due to right knee pain and decreased mobility. Previously the patient had a right total knee replacement for osteoarthritis. The patient also has extensive medical problems which were all monitored and treated while he was in the hospital: Parkinson's disease, hypertensive heart disease, congestive heart failure, bilateral capsular glaucoma, old MI six months ago, and recent abnormal cardiac stress test. Evaluation of the right knee indicated that patient had aseptic loosening of the tibial component of the knee. The orthopedic consultant indicated that the patient would need to be scheduled for a revision arthroplasty once he was cleared by cardiology for surgery. The cardiac clearance will be done as an outpatient and the procedure will then be scheduled. Assign the correct **diagnostic** code(s).

Code(s): _____

**1.221.** The patient is a 47-year-old-female admitted to the hospital for a scheduled total abdominal hysterectomy and bilateral salpingo-oophorectomy due to submucous leiomyoma of the uterus. The patient also has extensive endometriosis of the uterus, ovaries, and pelvic peritoneum. On the day of admission the patient was taken to surgery and in addition to the scheduled procedure lysis of extensive pelvic peritoneal adhesions was also carried out. In the process of removing the adhesions, the physician accidentally punctured the small bowel. This small puncture was quickly repaired. The patient was diagnosed with acute blood-loss anemia with a documented loss of 1,500 ml of blood during surgery. The remainder of the postoperative course was uneventful and the patient was discharged on day 4. Assign the **diagnosis** codes only.

Code(s): _____

> **Coding Guideline I.C.16.a.2. Principal Diagnosis for Birth Record**
> When coding the birth episode in a newborn record, assign a code from category, Z38, Liveborn infants according to the place of birth and type of delivery, as the principal diagnosis. A code from category Z38 is assigned only once, to a newborn at the time of birth. If a newborn is transferred to another institution, a code from category Z38 should not be used at the receiving hospital. A code from category Z38 is used only on the newborn record, not on the mother's record.

**1.222. Hospital Summary:** A male newborn, born at this hospital with pre-axial polydactyly of the thumbs and cleft deformities of both hands and feet, had a harsh murmur heard posteriorly and faint femoral pulses on initial newborn exam. The newborn was 39 weeks gestation and was born vaginally. Cardiology was consulted and an echocardiogram diagnosed coarctation of the aorta and a very small conoventricular ventricular septal defect. The newborn had surgical repair of the coarctation but the VSD could not be repaired at this young age due to closeness to the aortic valve. Cardiology will follow to manage the VSD. Orthopedics was consulted for the hand and feet deformities and will schedule serial repairs after the age of about 1 year. The family will be seen by Medical Genetics as an outpatient for possible determination of a syndrome that encompasses this combination of defects. Assign the correct **diagnostic** code(s).

Code(s): _____

# *Physician-Related Cases*

> **Coding Guideline IV.N. Ambulatory Surgery**
> For ambulatory surgery, code the diagnosis for which the surgery was performed. If the postoperative diagnosis is known to be different from the preoperative diagnosis at the time the diagnosis is confirmed, select the postoperative diagnosis for coding, since it is the most definitive.

**1.223.** The patient was seen with amenorrhea, characteristics of masculinization, and high levels of serum testosterone. Pelvic ultrasound revealed a left discrete ovarian mass. The GYN performed a laparoscopic unilateral salpingo-oophorectomy as an outpatient. Pathologic diagnosis returned as ovarian Sertoli-Leydig cell tumor. Upon receipt of the pathology report, what **diagnosis** does the GYN report?

Code(s): _____

**1.224.** The physician sees this 16-year-old patient with myasthenia gravis and adolescent idiopathic thoracic scoliosis. Surgery for spinal fusion was cancelled after the patient had a positive TB skin test during the preop physical workup, suggesting latent TB. On today's visit, the patient is started on Isoniazid 300 mg daily and instructed on possible side effects. She will reschedule surgery after two months of INH treatment. Assign the correct **diagnostic** code(s).

Code(s): _____

> **Coding Guideline IV.E. Encounters for Circumstances Other than a Disease or Injury**
> ICD-10-CM provides codes to deal with encounters for circumstances other than a disease or injury. The Factors Influencing Health Status and Contact with the Health Services codes (Z00-99) is provided to deal with occasions when circumstances other than a disease or injury are recorded as diagnosis or problems.

> **Coding Guideline I.C.21.c.2. Inoculations and Vaccinations**
> Code Z23 is for encounters for inoculations and vaccinations. It indicates that a patient is being seen to receive a prophylactic inoculation against a disease. Procedure codes are required to identify the actual administration of the injection and the type(s) of immunizations given. Code Z23 may be used as a secondary code if the inoculation is given as a routine part of preventive health care, such as a well-baby visit.

**1.225.** A 62-year-old female visits her family practice physician for an annual physical and follow-up on her chronic gout with tophi. She has her annual Pap smear and flu shot for the season. What **diagnoses** codes would the physician report?

Code(s): _____

**1.226.** The surgeon performed surgery on an 8-year-old boy who presented with progressive ataxia over a period of the past month. Surgical removal and frozen section identified the lesion as malignant ependymoma of the midbrain of the brain stem. During the surgical procedure, an accidental infratenorial intraoperative laceration left the patient with postsurgical left-sided muscle weakness and he will be sent for an outpatient rehabilitation evaluation next week. What code(s) would the surgeon submit for the case?

Code(s): _____

**1.227.** The following documentation is from the record of a 36-year-old male patient during a visit to his primary care physician.

**History of Present Illness:** The patient is here for follow-up of lab work from earlier in the week. He was bitten by a tick last month and has had body aches, some swelling to the right upper arm, pain and stiffness in the right elbow, as well as feeling fatigued. He had a Lyme test that came back positive and the patient is to have a repeat blood test today, the Western Blot test, as a secondary follow-up.

**Physical Examination:** He is alert and in no acute distress. Temp 98.4. Pulse 108. Respirations 20. Blood pressure is 118/70. Weight is 296 on a 5' 9" frame. Weight up 3 pounds from last week and 22 pounds up since the beginning of the year. Arm continues to display a circular erythematous lesion with 2+ pitting edema. The lesion has not grown outside the perimeter markings from his first visit.

**Impression:**
1. Localized arthritis, right elbow in Lyme disease due to tick bite
2. Morbid obesity, BMI of 43.7

The patient has blood drawn and was put on Doxycycline 100 mg b.i.d. × 4 weeks. Additional educational material on Lyme disease was given. He should follow-up immediately if the affected area grows larger than the current, marked area or if any new symptoms develop. We discussed again the need for an exercise program, when able, and portion control due to his over-nourishment status. Assign the correct **diagnostic** code(s).

Code(s): _____

**1.228.** The following documentation is from the office note of a podiatrist:

**S:** The patient presents for initial consult of tender lumps in the arches of both feet, left greater than right. Patient relates they have been present for several years and can change in size. Patient is also a diabetic and relates that his sugars are hard to control, running in the low 200s. Does get numbness in his feet.

**O:** Palpable pedal pulses bilaterally. Skin is warm with hair growth present. On plantar aspect of medial band of plantar fascia on the left, there is an approximately 1 × 1 cm elevated, solid lesion consistent with plantar fibroma. Pain with palpation. With palpation, medial band of plantar fascia on the right arch, there are two small, solid lesions noted, approximately 0.5 × 0.5 cm in diameter. These do not protrude through the skin as lesion on left foot does. Lesions on the right foot are nontender with palpation.

**A:** Plantar fibroma, bilateral, with left greater than right
Diabetes mellitus, type 2 with diabetic neuropathy

**P:** Discussed findings with patient. I advised that patient apply Triamcinolone cream to his feet to help decrease the size of the lesions. To help break down the lesion on the left arch, I injected 0.2 cc of 0.25% Marcaine plain and 0.2 cc of Kenalog into the lesion. The patient was instructed to work more diligently at controlling his sugars to prevent further neuropathy. I suggested Vitamin $B_6$ 200 mg and Vitamin $B_{12}$ 1,000 mcg, one tab of each daily to aid in nerve function. These are over the counter and can be purchased at the drug store. Patient is to follow-up with me in 4 to 6 weeks. Assign the correct **diagnostic** code(s).

Code(s): _____

**1.229.** The patient is a 42-year-old female with multiparity who presented for tubal ligation. She also had a large vulvar skin tag that the physician removed while the patient was under anesthesia. The physician listed diagnoses of multiparity, desiring sterilization by tubal ligation and vulvar skin tag, removed. What ICD-10-CM codes would the surgeon report?

Code(s): _____

**1.230.** The patient is a 49-year-old female with a chief complaint of painful mouth ulcers over the last month. She was treated with acyclovir for 10 days and penicillin on two occasions, including tapering doses of steroids on the second occasion. The patient states that she feels somewhat better but continues to have these ulcers with pain. Denies fever, chills, dysphagia, or lymphadenopathy. No high risk behavior.

**Physical Exam:** Reveals whitish patches measuring 1 mm × 1 mm on the buccal musoca and the hard palate. They are erythematous and inflamed.

**Assessment:** Aphthous ulcers and herpangina

**Plan:** Will start patient on clindamycin orally for buccal cellulitis and Amlexanox 5% as oral paste along with the Xylocaine mouth wash. Patient should follow up with me in 2 weeks. Assign the correct **diagnostic** code(s).

Code(s): _____

**1.231.** The patient was seen for menstrual irregularities, as well as new symptoms of vaginal itching and skin rash. The physician diagnoses vaginal candidiasis and tinea corporis on this visit, provides treatment as well as continuing treatment for the patient's polycystic ovarian syndrome. Assign the correct **diagnostic** code(s).

Code(s): _____

**1.232.** The patient presents for results of an MRI of the right knee, done to diagnose a new problem of severe pain and inability to safely descend stairs. She reports falling while running in the park. The MRI revealed a complex medial meniscal tear and a Baker's cyst, along with mild chondromalacia of the patella, which the physician discussed with the patient. Options for treatment were discussed and the patient will determine what she'd like to do, after discussing the situation with her husband and family. Assign the correct **diagnostic** code(s).

Code(s): _____

**1.233.** From a discharge summary written by an internal medicine physician:

The patient was admitted for dizziness and a vague feeling of epigastric discomfort. She has a history of duodenal carcinoma which was resected two years ago. The patient underwent chemo and has been in relatively good health over the last year until recently when she took a rapid decline. She no longer has evidence of an existing primary duodenal malignancy.

During her hospitalization, she underwent a GI workup to evaluate her current issues. An abdominal ultrasound showed a large liver mass. Oncology was consulted. The mass was further evaluated by needle biopsy and found to be metastatic carcinoma.

After lengthy consultation with me and the oncologist, the patient and family wish the patient to be a "Do Not Resuscitate" with no further workup and comfort care only. The patient was transferred from my service on the telemetry unit to the hospice program for ongoing palliative care.

What codes would the attending physician submit?

Code(s): _____

**1.234.** The following is taken from the records of a psychiatrist:

**Follow-up Visit:** The patient is a 10-year-old girl who is seen today to check progress after her Adderall XR was increased from 10 to 15 mg about six weeks ago. Since that time, the mother reports a very noticeable improvement in attention and task persistence, and a decrease in her hyperactivity and distractibility. This has also been commented on by her teacher and observed at home. She is now able to complete homework at one sitting, prior to dinner and without prompting. The teacher also reports less negativity than the patient had sometimes shown in the past.

**Status of Medication:** Adderall XR 15 mg with the above noted benefits. Appetite has been fine. Weight is stable.

**Vitals Signs:** Height 52½ inches, Weight 56.8 lbs, Blood pressure 96/54, Heart rate 91.

**Impression:** Medication showing clear benefits according to both teacher and parent.

**Diagnoses:**
Coordination disorder, developmental
Attention deficit disorder with hyperactivity, combined type

**Plan:** Continue current dosing. Three months of refills provided. Follow-up in three months. Assign the correct **diagnostic** code(s).

Code(s): _____

**1.235.** Reason for evaluation: Follow-up and medical management

**History:** The patient is a 5-year-old who has been in fairly good health. Her last skeletal dysplasia visit was 3 years ago. Since then, there has been some concern regarding signs of sleep apnea with a diagnosis of obstructive sleep apnea confirmed on sleep study. She has not had any imaging studies since her last visit.

The patient has a family history of achondroplasia in the father and the paternal grandmother. No other chromosomal abnormalities are noted. Her initial newborn bone survey showed bilateral foreshortening and splaying of the epiphyses of the distal and proximal ends of the femurs, irregular appearance of the developing acetabulum, thickening, with slight bowing of the femurs and lordosis. She has not reported any neurological issues and has never had a brain MRI. Her physical exam today is relatively unchanged and is remarkable for a large appearing head with frontal bossing, protuberant abdomen, lumbar hyperlordosis, extremity shortening with inability to extend elbow, trident-like hands and lax joints.

**Impression:**
1. Osteosclerosis congenita
2. Obstructive sleep apnea
3. Congenital lumbar lordosis
4. Family history of Osteosclerosis congenita

**Recommendations:** Weight management with dietitian to help prevent additional stress on bones and joints. Follow-up with me in one year. Assign the correct **diagnostic** code(s).

Code(s): _____

> **Coding Guideline IV.H. Uncertain Diagnosis**
> Do not code diagnoses documented as "probable," "suspected," "questionable," "rule out," or "working diagnosis" or other similar terms indicating uncertainty. Rather, code the condition(s) to the highest degree of certainty for that encounter/visit, such as symptoms, signs, abnormal test results, or other reasons for the visit.

**1.236.** From the record of a primary care physician:

**Chief complaint:** Vertigo

**HPI:** The patient is a 55-year-old Caucasian female who presents with vertigo over the last month. She has had vertigo symptoms mostly when lying down on her back. She gets a dizzy feeling which she describes as spinning and reports some decreased hearing and buzzing in the left ear. Symptoms last about 30 minutes, relieved when she does not move. She denies nausea, vomiting, or any other neurologic symptoms associated with this dizziness. She also describes left-sided temporal pain which she states feels like she is going to develop a headache but never quite develops into a headache. It comes and goes many times throughout the day.

**Past Medical History:** None

**Review of Systems:** As above

**Physical Exam:** She is afebrile. Vital signs are stable. Neurologic exam is unremarkable. Cerebellar exam is normal. PERRLA. EOM intact. No nystagmus with lateral gaze. Vision is WNL on screening with no diplopia. Tympanic membranes are normal ×2. Posterior pharynx is normal. Neck is supple. No lymphadenopathy. No rigidity. Lungs are clear to auscultation bilaterally. Heart is regular rate and rhythm without murmur. Normal S1, S2. Abdomen: Soft and nontender. Extremities: No edema. Skin: without rash or significant lesions. No tenderness over the temporal artery. Neuro: Cranial nerves II-XII are intact.

**Assessment and Plan:**
1. Labyrinthine vertigo. Patient agrees to PT evaluation. Will try Antivert for spinning.
2. Headache with normal neurologic exam. ESR ordered to rule out temporal arteritis due to the location.

Patient to return in two weeks for follow-up. Assign the correct **diagnostic** code(s).

Code(s): _____

**1.237.** From the clinic record of a family practice physician:

**Problem:** Hospital Follow-up

**S:** The patient is here for follow-up of new diagnosis of Bell's palsy, made during hospitalization over the weekend. He thought he was having a stroke but complete evaluation ruled out stroke and diagnosed Bell's palsy. He was started on medication for this. His main concern today is a lot of ear pain and jaw pain on the left that have been increasing since his discharge on Monday. He describes the jaw pain as burning and stinging in nature.

**O:** Patient is in no acute distress but is obviously in some pain. Vital signs are stable. Left TM is erythematous. Right TM is gray. He does have a notable Bell's palsy with the droop of his face on the left as well as persistent inability to close the left eyelid. Palpation of the jaw area elicits a hot, shooting pain. Lungs are clear. Cardiovascular reveals regular rate and rhythm.

**A:** Bell's palsy. New facial pain, rule out superimposed trigeminal neuralgia. Nonsuppurative otitis media.

**P:** I did start him on Bactrim double strength dose twice a day for 10 days. I have recommended Tylenol for pain. He should continue to use the eyedrops prescribed by the neurologist and I gave him an eye patch to use at nighttime to rest the eye. I have arranged another appointment for later today with the neurologist to further evaluate the increasing jaw pain and recommend treatment. Follow-up with me as necessary.

Assign the correct **diagnostic** code(s).

Code(s): _____

**1.238.** The patient is a 54-year-old female who presents today with an infected cuticle on her left thumbnail. The patient states this started about one week ago. She denies any discharge from the nail but throbbing pain at night. She does work as a bartender where she is frequently having her hands immersed in water. She denies any trauma to her hand. No possibility of a fracture. No nausea, vomiting or diarrhea, fever or chills. The patient does have a cough. She is a smoker for the past 20+ years. She smokes a pack of cigarettes a day. The cough is typical and sometimes productive of whitish clear sputum.

**Allergies:** Penicillin and iodine both which produce hives.

**Social History:** Admits to drinking two beers a day. No illicit drug use.

**Review of Systems:** The patient has never had a chest x-ray done. She is up to date on her Pap smears and mammogram.

**Physical Exam:** Blood pressure is 118/66. Pulse 70. Respiration 12. Temp is 98.5. Lungs are clear to auscultation. No rales, rhonchi, or wheezing. Heart is RRR. Abdomen is soft, nontender, and nondistended. To the lateral aspect of the left thumbnail bed there is increased swelling and erythema with no discharge noted. There is exquisite tenderness on palpation.

**Impression:**
1. Paronychia left thumbnail - levaquin 750 mg once a day for five days
2. Smokers' cough - chest x-ray ordered, CMP, lipids, TSH and CBC ordered.
3. Tobacco abuse

Assign the correct **diagnostic** code(s).

Code(s): _____

> **Coding Guideline I.C.15.a.1. Codes from Chapter 15 and Sequencing Priority**
> Obstetrics cases require codes from Chapter 15, codes in the range of O00-O9A, Pregnancy, childbirth and the puerperium. Chapter 15 codes have sequencing priority over codes from other chapters. Additional codes from other chapters may be used in conjunction with Chapter 15 codes to further specify conditions. Should the provider document that the pregnancy is incidental to the encounter, then code Z33.1, Pregnant state, incidental, should be used in place of any Chapter 15 codes. It is the provider's responsibility to state that the condition being treated is not affecting the pregnancy.

**1.239.** The patient is a 32-year-old female with Hashimoto thyroiditis and gestational diabetes, currently 34 weeks gestation. She is seen for ongoing monitoring of the conditions. Blood sugars and thyroid lab results are reviewed. Synthroid is increased to 0.125 mg p.o. daily. The endocrinologist will see her back six weeks postpartum to re-evaluate her conditions. The endocrinologist documents the following diagnoses: Hashimoto thyroiditis complicating pregnancy and gestational diabetes, well controlled utilizing dietary measures. Assign the correct **diagnostic** code(s).

Code(s): _____

**1.240.** The following documentation is from the health record of a 25-year-old female patient.

**History of Present Illness:** The patient is a Caucasian female without significant medical history and is 18 weeks pregnant. She presents with a 6-month history of right hand pain and paresthesias, happening prior to her pregnancy. This seems to be worse over the last 1 month. She states that she bought a hand splint for nighttime but typing and writing during the day makes it hurt significantly. She says she's always had cold hands/fingertips. When she runs them under warm water, this improves them. She denies any color changes in the fingertips. The paresthesias seem to involve most of the fingers. The pain seems to be mostly in the palm of the hand. The only relieving factors are heating her hand.

**Past Surgical History:** None.
**Medications:** Prenatal vitamins.
**Allergies:** No known drug allergies.
**Family History:** No neurological issues.

**Physical Examination:** On exam, her blood pressure is 122/68. Pulse is 82. Both her hands are warm. Right fingertips are considerably cooler. There are no color changes. She has good distal pulses. Hands are neurovascularly intact. There is no thenar atrophy. Strength is 5/5 in the fingers and wrists. Phalen and Tinel sign are negative. Skin has no rashes.

**Assessment and Plan:** Right hand pain and paresthesias. Incidental pregnancy. She should wear her right wrist splint at night and in the day as tolerated. She will get an ergonomic keyboard. She will take Tylenol for pain and avoid all other analgesics due to pregnancy. She will have a TSH to rule out hypothyroidism and will have right upper extremity EMG/nerve conduction. If this is normal, we could consider the possibility of Raynaud phenomenon. She will follow up with me after her testing is complete. Assign the correct **diagnostic** code(s).

Code(s): _____

**1.241.** The following is an admission H&P dictated by the patient's primary care provider:

**Reason for Admission:** Malaise, low-grade fever, and diarrhea

**HPI:** This is a 60-year-old male with severe peripheral vascular disease who had recently been hospitalized for C. difficile diarrhea, which seemed to resolve well with treatment. His diarrhea was basically resolved after his 5-day admission. He went home and was doing fine but over the last week he started developing more malaise, low-grade fever and the watery and frequent diarrhea returned. He presented to the ED today and was admitted.

**Past Medical History:** He has peripheral vascular disease of both lower legs. He also has had a peptic ulcer in the remote past.

**Social History:** He lives at home with his wife and does have a supportive family. He does not smoke or drink.

**Physical Exam:** His blood pressure is low at 90/60. His temperature is 97.2. HEENT: Pupils are equal and reactive to light and accommodation. There is some weakness of an ocular muscle. Neck: Supple. Lungs: Clear. Heart: S1 and S2. No murmur. No gallop. Abdomen: There is some minimal diffuse tenderness to his abdomen on palpation. Extremities: No edema or cyanosis in the thighs. The lower legs are both looking better than on past admission.

**Impression:** Recurrence of Clostridium difficile colitis.

**Plan:** Started on flagyl and vancomycin. C. diff cultures will be obtained. We will also check blood cultures and urine cultures. The patient is dehydrated and IV fluids started in the ED will be continued. Will ask Vascular to consult about the need for DVT prophylaxis due to decreased mobility while hospitalized.

What codes should the physician report?

Code(s): _____

**1.242.** Primary care provider note from the record of a 44-year-old female patient:

**CC:** Mourning
**History:** The patient is here because of fatigue. Does not want to get out of bed, is still crying and wants to give up on her life. The patient did see a counselor for one visit a couple of months ago but she says it didn't really help. She has not been feeling any better and is depressed. She is eating appropriately and is well groomed today. She denies any serious suicidal ideation.

**Physical Exam:** She is 44 and weighs 151 pounds. She is 5 feet tall. Blood pressure is 112/60. HEENT is WNL. Lungs are clear. Heart is regular rate and rhythm. Abdomen: Benign.

**Assessment and Plan:** Major depression with bereavement of husband. She was given fluoxetine 10 mg daily for a week, then 20 mg daily for a week. She is to return to the office to see me in 2 weeks. Assign the correct **diagnostic** code(s).

Code(s): _____

**1.243.** This 30-year-old male patient has exhausted all types of conservative treatment for his morbid obesity. Despite regular consultation with a registered dietitian, he continues to eat in excess of 7,000 calories per day. This may be attributed to his very low-literacy level. He has been treated in this clinic for the last three years. He has also been treated for hypertension and hypercholesterolemia. With these risk factors and with careful review of his condition and symptoms and with consultation regarding the risks and benefits of surgery, it has been decided to perform a vertical-banded gastroplasty two weeks from this office visit. Assign the correct **diagnostic** code(s).

Code(s): _____

---

**Coding Note:** When coding otitis media, ICD-10-CM provides laterality specificity at the sixth character level.

---

**1.244.** From the clinic record of a family practice physician:

**Subjective:** The patient is a 12-month-old female patient who presents to the clinic today with a possible ear infection. She has been waking up at night and is irritable. She has had some cold-like symptoms as well as some purulent drainage from her eyes over the past four days. She has had a fever since last night. This morning the temperature is back to near normal. No cough and appetite has been slightly decreased.

**Objective:** In no acute distress; alert and interactive. Temperature is 100.7.

**HEENT:** Lids and sclera are normal. No erythema noted. She does have some purulent drainage mostly on the left lower lid. She also has a purulent nasal discharge that is yellow to green. TMs are erythematous bilaterally, bulging and with purulent effusions. Oropharynx is nonerythematous without lesions. Tonsils are unremarkable. Two teeth on the bottom.

**Neck:** Neck is supple with good ROM. Positive cervical adenopathy.
**Lungs:** Clear.
**Heart:** Regular rate and rhythm without murmur.

**Assessment:**
1. Acute bilateral suppurative otitis media
2. Upper respiratory infection

**Plan:** The patient will be placed on Augmentin 40 mg/kg. divided t.i.d. for 10 days. Also recommended lots of fluids and rest, decongestants and elevating the head of the bed for symptomatic control. I believe the eyes are due to backup from her nose and not due to conjunctivitis at this point. The parents will need to contact the clinic if she develops any erythema or persistent drainage. The parents are comfortable with this plan and will contact the clinic with any further questions and/or concerns. Assign the correct **diagnostic** code(s).

Code(s): _____

> **Coding Note:** ICD-10-CM provides combination codes that include the type of diabetes mellitus and the manifestation/complication.

> **Coding Note:** The Tabular instructs the coding professional to use an additional code with type 2 diabetes to identify any insulin use.

**1.245.** Assign the code(s) for a patient with type 2 diabetic gastroparesis who is presently on insulin.

Code(s): _____

**1.246.** A 20-year-old patient with end-stage renal disease is seen for monitoring of his condition. The patient is currently receiving dialysis three times a week. He has an A-V fistula in his left arm for vascular access. Assign the correct **diagnostic** code(s).

Code(s): _____

> **Coding Guideline I.C.21.c.8. Follow-up**
> The follow-up codes are used to explain continuing surveillance following complete treatment of a disease, condition, or injury. A follow-up code may be used to explain multiple visits. Should a condition be found to have recurred on the follow-up visit, then the diagnosis code for the condition should be assigned in place of the follow-up code.

**1.247.** From the health records of a patient receiving endoscopy services:

The patient presents to the hospital outpatient department for follow-up cystoscopy for a history of high-grade bladder cancer. This was resected five years ago and was found to be Grade III with superficial muscle invasion. A cycle of chemotherapy was provided, but no radiation. No recurrence has been noted since then. CT scan of the pelvis six months ago was negative for masses. Sometimes the patient experiences painful ejaculation, but no hematospermia has been found. Cytology to date has been negative.

Cystoscopy examination today shows a new primary site of transitional cell carcinoma of the anterior wall of the bladder. There is some lateral lobe prostatic hypertrophy, just barely touching in the midline. The bladder is nontrabeculated. There is clear efflux from each orifice. The area of resection was around the right ureteral orifice, which appears a little atrophic, but patent. Patient is scheduled for surgery as soon as convenient.

**Impression:** Stable transitional cell carcinoma of the bladder with mild benign prostatic hypertrophy. Assign the correct **diagnostic** code(s).

Code(s): _____

**1.248.** This 70-year-old patient is seen for his follow-up care for his arthritis. He has primary generalized degenerative arthritis mostly of the knees, hip, and of the lumbosacral spine. It is getting progressively worse. He refuses surgery and is not a prime candidate because of his arteriosclerotic heart disease and hypertension. A prescription was written to renew his Celebrex and other medications for his ASHD and hypertension. Assign the correct **diagnostic** code(s).

Code(s): _____

**1.249.** A 13-year-old male patient is being evaluated in the Children's Clinic for growth problems. He is 4'11" and does not exhibit any signs of puberty or secondary sexual characteristics. His parents wonder if the necrotizing enterocolitis that he had at birth is the cause of his short stature. Other than his short stature, the patient seems perfectly normal. His short stature does create problems at school, however, as he is experiencing definite problems with social rejection and exclusion because of his height. Blood tests were drawn. Diagnosis: Short stature with delayed puberty.

The patient came back to the clinic for follow-up of test results, which indicated a deficiency of growth hormone. The patient was started on growth hormone treatments. Diagnosis on the second visit is HGH deficiency. Provide the ICD-10-CM codes for both the first and second visit. Assign the correct **diagnostic** code(s).

Code(s) for first visit: _____

Code(s) for second visit: _____

**Coding Note:** In ICD-10-CM, when coding an infection due to an indwelling urinary catheter, the coding professional is instructed to use an additional code to identify the infection. Additionally, if the infectious agent is also known, this should be assigned as an additional diagnosis.

**1.250.** A nursing home patient with an indwelling Foley catheter is diagnosed at the physician office, with a serious urinary tract infection due to E. coli caused by the catheter. The catheter is removed and a urine culture and sensitivity is sent. The catheter is replaced through the urethra, and aggressive antibiotic therapy is begun. The patient is returned to the nursing home for continued follow-up. Assign the correct **diagnostic** code(s).

Code(s): _____

**Coding Guideline I.C.9.a.3. Hypertensive Heart and Chronic Kidney Disease**
Assign codes from combination category I13, Hypertensive heart and chronic kidney disease, when both hypertensive kidney disease and hypertensive heart disease are stated in the diagnosis. Assume a relationship between the hypertension and the chronic kidney disease, whether or not the condition is so designated. If heart failure is present, assign an additional code from category I50 to identify the type of heart failure. The appropriate code from category N18, Chronic kidney disease, should be used as a secondary code with a code from category I13 to identify the stage of the chronic kidney disease.

**1.251.** A patient is seen in the hospital with a diagnosis of congestive heart failure due to hypertensive heart disease. The patient responds positively to Lasix therapy. The patient also has chronic kidney disease stage 5. Assign the correct **diagnostic** codes.

Code(s): _____

# *Hospital Outpatient Cases*

---

**Coding Guideline I.C.1.a.2.d. Asymptomatic Immunodeficiency Virus**
Z21, Asymptomatic human immunodeficiency virus [HIV] infection status, is to be applied when the patient without any documentation of symptoms is listed as being "HIV positive," "known HIV," "HIV test positive," or similar terminology. Do not use this code if the term "AIDS" is used or if the patient is treated for any HIV-related illness or is described as having any condition(s) resulting from his/her HIV positive status; use B20 in these cases.

---

**Coding Guideline IV.H. Uncertain Diagnosis for Outpatient Services**
Do not code diagnoses documented as "probable," "suspected," "questionable," "rule out," or "working diagnosis" or other similar terms indicating uncertainty. Rather, code the condition(s) to the highest degree of certainty for that encounter/visit, such as symptoms, signs, abnormal test results, or other reason for the visit.

---

**1.252.** The following documentation is from the health record of a male patient who received emergency department services.

**Emergency Department Report**
A patient, who is a known heroin addict, is brought into the emergency room in significant distress. His genitalia are covered with many lesions. Due to his IV drug habit and sexual practices, he is at risk for HIV exposure and hepatitis. He is unable to provide a medical history, but the physician is able to get some information from his girlfriend. Although severely ill, he is not comatose.

Physical examination reveals multiple excoriations covering the penis and scrotum with fluid-filled blisters and the patient is in significant distress. The patient is heavily intoxicated and the last "fix" was one hour ago per the girlfriend. The patient has been using heroin daily for the past two months. A number of laboratory tests were run, and it was determined that the patient should be transferred to a tertiary care center for definitive treatment with an infectious disease consultation and substance abuse rehabilitation when stable.

The physician's dictated report that details the test results shows the following diagnostic assessment:
1. HSV-2 infection, culture confirmed, severe outbreak
2. Hepatitis suspected, pending laboratory results for type, abnormal liver function studies confirmed
3. HIV seropositive
4. High-risk lifestyle; sexual habits and drug addict
5. Heroin intoxication

Assign the correct **diagnostic** code(s).

Code(s): _____

**1.253.** The encounter is to receive chemotherapy following the recent diagnosis of carcinoma of the pancreas neck. The cancer was diagnosed two months ago and the patient has been receiving chemotherapy. After the chemotherapy administration, the patient developed severe nausea and vomiting due to the chemotherapy, which led to dehydration. Medications were given for the nausea and vomiting. IV fluids were given to rehydrate the patient. What **diagnosis** codes are assigned?

Code(s): _____

---

**Coding Guideline I.C.18.b. Use of a Symptom Code with a Definitive Diagnosis Code**
Signs or symptoms that are associated routinely with a disease process should not be assigned as additional codes, unless otherwise instructed by the classification.

---

**1.254.** The following documentation is from the health record of a 39-year-old male patient.

**Emergency Department Services**
**History of Present Illness:** The patient is a 39-year-old African-American gentleman who has a known history of sickle-cell Hb-C disease who presented to the Emergency Department with diffuse extremity pains with a little more complaints of pain along the right inguinal area. They started on Friday, became a little bit better on Saturday, then improved; and again started in the past 24 hours. He denies any problems with cough or sputum or production. He denies any problems with fever.

**Past Medical History:** See recent medical records in charts. He does have a new onset of diabetes, probably related to his hemochromatosis. He does have evidence of iron overload with high ferritins.

**Review of Systems:** Otherwise unremarkable except for those related to his pain. He denies any problems with any fever or night sweats. No cough or sputum production. Denies any changes in gastrointestinal or genitourinary habits. No blood per rectum or urine.

**Physical Examination:** This is a 39-year-old African-American gentleman who is conscious and cooperative. He is oriented ×3 and appears in no acute distress. Vital signs are stable. HEENT is remarkable for icterus present in oral mucosa and conjunctivae, which is a chronic event for him. The neck is supple. No evidence of any gross lymphadenopathy of the cervical, supraclavicular, or axillary areas. The heart is irregular in rate without any murmurs heard. Lungs are clear to auscultation and percussion. The abdomen is soft and benign without any gross organomegaly. Extremities reveal no edema. No palpable cords. He does have some tenderness along the inner aspects of his right lower extremity near the inguinal area; however, no masses were palpable and no point tenderness is noted.

IV fluids and pain medications were administered in the ED. He had a problem with his right inguinal area. He had evidence of pain. There was some pain on abduction of his right lower extremity. The wrist really was unremarkable. There was no evidence of any Holman, no palpable cords, no masses were palpable.

Because of his sickle-cell anemia, rule out the possibility of avascular necrosis of the femur. Complete x-rays of his femur and hip were carried out. However, these were both negative.

Patient is being transferred to a larger facility for treatment of his sickle-cell crisis. Unfortunately, he has very little family support with his medical issues. Doppler studies should also be carried out to rule out any venous thrombosis.

**Diagnoses:**
1. Painful sickle-cell crisis
2. Type 2 diabetes mellitus
3. Limited family support

**Condition on Discharge:** Stable on pain meds.

Assign the correct **diagnostic** code(s).

Code(s): _____

**1.255.** The following documentation is from the health record of a 66-year-old male patient.

**Outpatient Hospital Department Services**
**History:** This is a 66-year-old gentleman who had coronary artery bypass graft two months ago and continues to do well. Sometime after he was discharged home, he had two days of black stools. He has not had any other evidence of hematemesis, melena, or hematochezia but was feeling rather weak and fatigued. He had blood work done which showed a hemoglobin of 9.7, hematocrit of 20.9, MCV of 80 and serum iron of 8.2% saturation. No indigestion, heartburn, or abdominal pain of any kind. There is no past history of anemia or GI bleed.

**Past Medical History:** General health has been good.
**Allergies:** None known
**Previous Surgeries:** Coronary artery bypass graft
**Medications:** At the time of admission include Glucotrol, Lasix, and potassium

**Review of Systems:** Endocrine: He does have diabetes, controlled with oral medication. Cardiovascular: Coronary artery disease with coronary artery bypass graft. No recent symptoms of chest pain or shortness of breath. Respiratory: No chronic cough or sputum production. GU: No dysuria, hematuria, history of stones, or infections. Musculoskeletal: No arthritic complaints or muscle weakness. Neuropsychiatric: No syncope, seizures, weakness, paralysis, depression.

**Family History:** Is positive for cardiovascular disease and diabetes in his mother. No history of cancer.

**Social History:** The patient is married. Has never smoked and does not drink. Works in a factory where he is exposed to high levels of industrial toxic agents.

Physical examination reveals a well-developed, well-nourished, alert male in no acute distress. Blood pressure: 146/82. Respirations: 18. Heart rate: 78. Skin: Good turgor and texture. Eyes: No scleral icterus. Pupils are round, regular, equal, and react to light. Neck: No jugular venous distention. No carotid bruits. Thyroid is not enlarged. Trachea is in the midline. Lungs are clear. Heart: No murmur noted. Abdomen is soft. Bowel sounds present. No masses, no tenderness. Liver and spleen are not palpably enlarged. Extremities: Good pulses. Trace edema of the feet.

Laboratory values show severe anemia with a hemoglobin of 9.7. His iron studies showed low iron and low ferritin, consistent with chronic blood loss anemia. His $B_{12}$ and folate levels were normal. His SMA-12 was essentially unremarkable.

**Recommendations:** Patient should have an esophagogastroduodenoscopy and colonoscopy, possible biopsy or polypectomy, as well as a blood transfusion, which has been explained to the patient along with potential risks and complications. These will be scheduled as soon as possible.

**Final Diagnoses:**
1. Severe blood loss anemia; weakness
2. Type 2 diabetes mellitus
3. Coronary artery disease status post coronary artery bypass graft
4. Unhealthy work environment

The patient was scheduled for EGD and colonoscopy as well as a blood transfusion. The patient will be discharged home and he will have clear liquid diet. He is to call for any problems. He will continue with his home medications, and he was placed on ferrous sulfate 1 tablet twice a day. Assign the correct **diagnostic** code(s).

Code(s): _____

**1.256.** The following documentation is from the health record of a 2-week-old baby.

**Emergency Department Services**
A 2-week-old baby is rushed to the hospital after the parents checked and found her cyanotic. While in the ER, she suffered respiratory arrest followed by cardiac arrest and was given cardiopulmonary resuscitation. The baby was born with a birth weight of 2,400 g. Her current weight is 2,700 g. The baby was emergently transferred to the neonatal intensive care unit at the university hospital across town for monitoring and further workup. Final diagnosis for the ER service is "Hypoxia with respiratory failure in a low birth weight infant—etiology unknown." Assign the correct **diagnostic** code(s).

Code(s): _____

**1.257.** The following documentation is from the health record of a 51-year-old female patient:
**Emergency Department Services**
The patient has a history of serious illnesses, including type 1 diabetic complications, that include severe peripheral vascular disease of the extremities. She presented to the ER via ambulance with chest pain and shortness of breath.

She has been hypertensive for many years and is currently well controlled on medication. Her BP in the ER was stable but was monitored frequently. The patient's blood sugar was also monitored.

**Impression:**
Chest pain and shortness of breath
Rule out CHF vs. pulmonary embolus
Diabetes mellitus, type 1, out of control, with significant peripheral vascular disease

**Plan:** Transfer to University Hospital.

Assign the correct **diagnostic** code(s).

Code(s): _____

---

**Coding Guideline I.C.20.k. External Cause Status**

A code from category Y99, External cause status, should be assigned whenever any other external cause code is assigned for an encounter, including an activity code, except for the events noted below. Assign a code from category Y99, External cause status, to indicate the work status of the person at the time the event occurred. The status code indicates whether the event occurred during military activity, whether a non-military person was at work, whether an individual including a student or volunteer was involved in a non-work activity at the time of the causal event.

A code from Y99, External cause status, should be assigned, when applicable, with other external cause codes, such as transport accidents and falls. The external cause status codes are not applicable to poisonings, adverse effects, misadventures, or late effects.

Do not assign a code from category Y99 if no other external cause codes (cause, activity) are applicable for the encounter.

An external cause status code is used only once, at the initial encounter for treatment. Only one code from Y99 should be recorded on a medical record.

Do not assign code Y99.9, Unspecified external cause status, if the status is not stated.

---

**1.258.** The patient is seen in the ER today for a burn of the right ankle. The patient was cooking dinner in the kitchen of her single family home and carrying a pot of boiling hot liquid that splashed on her ankle. The physician documents the diagnosis as: Second degree burn, right ankle. Assign the correct **diagnostic** code(s).

Code(s): _____

**1.259.** The following documentation is from the health record of a male patient who received emergency department services.

**Emergency Department Report:** This is a 48-year-old male patient who presents to the ED with a history of left lower quadrant abdominal pain for two days. The patient has localized tenderness with some guarding on the left lower quadrant.

**Past Medical History:** Hypertension
**Past Surgical History:** Right rotator cuff surgery
**Allergies:** Ibuprofen
**Medications:** Diovan HCT
**Social History:** Patient smokes cigarettes, alcohol socially
**Family History:** Father had diverticulitis and cancer of the colon

**Review of Systems:** Negative nausea, vomiting, or diarrhea. Had a relatively normal bowel movement earlier today. No rectal bleeding. All other systems reviewed and are negative.

**Physical Examination:** No acute distress but in pain. Vital signs: Temp is 98.6, pulse 88, respirations 20, blood pressure 116/78. HEENT: Within normal limits. Neck: Supple, no masses, no bruit. Heart: Regular S1, S2 present. No chest pain. Lungs: Clear. No shortness of breath, no cough. Abdomen: Soft. Tenderness with guarding of the left lower quadrant. Bowel sounds are present. Extremities: No calf tenderness. Pulses are palpable. Sensory motor system is intact. Neurological: Patient is alert and oriented.

A stat CBC was done which showed white cell count of 20,000.

**Impression:**
1. Acute diverticulitis
2. Family history of colon cancer
3. Hypertension

The patient is started on Levaquin and Flagyl and will continue his at-home hypertension med. A surgical consult is requested and the surgeon recommended admission to 23-hour observation. Assign the correct **diagnostic** code(s).

Code(s): _____

**1.260.** The patient presented to the hospital urgent-care center, complaining of a swollen left upper eyelid for the past 2 days. She stated that the swelling was increasing and putting more and more pressure on her eye. The eyelashes were affecting her vision as the angle of the lashes had changed due to the swelling. She reported a history of surgery to her sinus on the left side about 2 months ago. On physical exam the physician noted that the left eyelid and surrounding tissue was severely swollen and had a focal area consistent with an internal hordeolum.

The assessment was internal hordeolum of left eyelid with secondary orbital cellulitis and the physician prescribed Keflex 500 mg 4 times a day for 7 days and cortisporin ophthalmic ointment twice daily to the eye. The physician advised washing the eyelid with Johnson's No More Tears baby shampoo twice daily, using good handwashing technique and not touching either eye during the healing process, except for treatments as above. The patient was told to follow up with her PMD in 3 days for a recheck or sooner if the area increases in size. Assign the correct **diagnostic** code(s).

Code(s): _____

**1.261.** The following documentation is from the health record of a female patient who received emergency department services.

**Emergency Department Report**
**Chief Complaint:** Multiple Sclerosis

**S:** The patient presents today with numbness and pain in her left arm and leg and in her back. She says it feels the way it felt when she was first diagnosed with MS several years ago. She came in today because of a rather sharp pain over her lungs and in her chest area while she was driving to work. She came here rather than continuing on to work. She describes the pain as fairly sharp and stabbing. It was exacerbated when she took a deeper breath, which really scared her. She denies any coughing with this and she denies any diaphoresis with it.

**O:** Patient is in mild distress and is breathing rather shallowly to avoid pain. Her BP is 126/78, pulse 88, respirations 24. Temp is 99.3 degrees. Lungs: Essentially clear. CV: Regular rate and rhythm and no murmurs. Extremities: without edema. EKG is unchanged from previous and chest x-ray shows blunting in the costophrenic angle but no infiltrates or pneumothorax seen.

**A:** Exacerbation of multiple sclerosis with viral pleurisy.

**P:** The patient will start Prednisone 60 mg a day with the tapering schedule to be determined by the neurologist at her outpatient evaluation the day after tomorrow. She will begin Indomethacin 25 mg twice a day and will take Tylenol if additional pain relief is needed. The patient is placed off of work and will avoid any strenuous activity. She should return if her symptoms get worse or for additional pain management if a cough develops. Assign the correct **diagnostic** code(s).

Code(s): _____

> **Coding Guideline I.C.13.a. Site and Laterality**
> Most of the codes within Chapter 13 have site and laterality designations. The site represents either the bone, joint, or the muscle involved. For some conditions where more than one bone, joint, or muscle is usually involved, such as osteoarthritis, there is a "multiple sites" code available. For categories where no multiple site code is provided and more than one bone, joint, or muscle is involved, multiple codes should be used to indicate the different sites involved.

**1.262.** The following documentation is from the health record of a female patient who is receiving care from the Rheumatology Clinic.

**Follow-up Clinic Note**

**HPI:** The patient returns now for a follow-up visit. She has been on Plaquenil for about 6 weeks. Overall she feels somewhat better. She does report a new issue with incontinence and wonders if this is related to either of her medications. She describes this as an urgency and as leakage if she sneezes or coughs. She seems to otherwise be tolerating her medications without difficulty.

**Physical Exam:** Examination today shows her vital signs to be stable. She is afebrile. Joints show inflammation in the right ankle and left wrist. The remainder of the upper and lower extremity joints are quiet.

**Impression:** Palindromic rheumatism on methotrexate and Plaquenil. Urge and stress incontinence.

**Plan:** UA done in the office today is normal. Review of medication literature does not give any evidence that either medication is associated with urinary incontinence. I recommended that she make an appointment with the Urology clinic to discuss this new issue. The patient and I again talked about the need to avoid methotrexate in situations where she could become dehydratd because of potential renal clearance problems. She was instructed not to take methotrexate if she has been vomiting for more than 12 hours without consultation here. The patient will have a hemogram, liver function panel, and creatinine today and then will follow up with this clinic in 8 weeks. If she has other illnesses, she will call us, hold her methotrexate and arrange to be seen either here or in the emergency department for evaluation. Assign the correct **diagnostic** code(s).

Code(s): _____

**1.263.** The following documentation is the discharge note of a female patient who received emergency department and observation services.

**HPI:** The patient presents today with blurred vision which resolved after a duration of 20 minutes, left temporal headache, and left lower extremity weakness and numbness. The lower extremity complaints resolved within the first hour in the ED. She states that the headache has been an 8 or 9 out of 10 but her vision has improved. She recalls headaches like this in the past but not this painful and without the associated symptoms.

**Vitals Signs:** In the ED, her blood pressure was 143/88, pulse 80, respirations 20, temperature 97.4. HEENT: all within normal limits. Chest: Clear to auscultation bilaterally. Cardiac: Normal S1, S2. Slight bradycardia. No heaves, murmurs, or rubs. Abdomen: Soft. Nontender. No HSM. Extremities. No clubbing, cyanosis, or edema. Sensation has completely returned. Gait is now normal. Neurological: Cranial nerves II-XII are intact. Alert and oriented ×3. The patient was admitted to 23 hour observation for intractable headache.

**Observation Course:** The patient was seen by neurology and an MRI, 2D echo, ESR, and RPR were all checked. Her results were essentially negative. CT scan showed no bleed, no mass effect or shift. Her carotid dopplers were within normal limits. MRI showed no acute infarct but some small vessel ischemic changes. The patient was also seen by cardiology and was cleared by them. Her EKG showed signs of bradycardia and her 2D echo was normal.

Pain was managed with morphine 2.5–4mg IV q 6–8hrs with resolution at approximately observation hour number 14. The patient was discharged on no medication and will follow up with neurology as an outpatient.

**Impression:** Cluster headache, intractable. Secondary cause ruled out. Assign the correct **diagnostic** code.

Code(s): _____

> **Coding Guideline IV.A.2. Observation Stay**
> When a patient is admitted for observation for a medical condition, assign a code for the medical condition as the first-listed diagnosis.
>
> When a patient presents for outpatient surgery and develops complications requiring admission to observation, code the reason for the surgery as the first reported diagnosis (reason for the encounter), followed by codes for the complications as secondary diagnoses.

> **Coding Guideline I.C.21.c.9. Donor**
> Codes in category Z52, Donors of organs or tissues, are used for living individuals who are donating blood or other body tissue. These codes are only for individuals donating for others, not for self-donations. They are not used to identify cadaveric donations.

**1.264.** This 24-year-old male bone marrow donor was taken to the Same Day Surgery suite and, under general anesthesia, 200 cc of bone marrow was aspirated from the posterior iliac crests. During postop recovery, the patient developed a postop fever, nausea, and vomiting and was subsequently admitted to observation. The nausea and vomiting subsided following medication. The patient became afebrile and was discharged home. Assign the correct **diagnostic** code(s).

Code(s): _____

**1.265.** The patient is taken to the outpatient surgical suite for an ERCP to remove a stone from the common bile duct. The patient has a history of tachycardia which recurred after the procedure. The patient was admitted to observation until the heart rate could be stabilized.

**Preoperative Diagnosis:** Jaundice due to calculus obstruction of the common bile duct

**Postoperative Diagnosis:** Jaundice due to calculus obstruction of the common bile duct, tachycardia. Assign the correct **diagnostic** code(s).

Code(s): _____

**1.266.** The patient is a 1Y, 11M old female who presents to the emergency department with a 2-day history of pain in the left groin area. Four months ago, the patient had a similar problem on the right side and was diagnosed with an inguinal fold abscess. She has no fever today, is on no medication, and does have an allergy to Bactrim, which was tried last time.

On examination, the patient has a 2 cm × 1 cm abscess of the left labia majora toward the inguinal fold. Yellow pus was expressed and there is no surrounding erythema. The remainder of the exam was normal.

Findings are a nearly 2-year-old female with labial abscess from what appears to be staph. The patient is given Keflex 250 mg/5 ml, 4 ml PO TID × 10 days and Bactroban BID × 5 days. The mother is to clean the area with Hibaclens at every diaper change. Follow-up with the PMD in 1 week or sooner if fever, increased erythema, or rash. Assign the correct **diagnostic** code(s).

Code(s): _____

**1.267.** The following documentation is from the health record of a female patient who received emergency department services.

**Emergency Department Report**

The patient presents to the emergency department today complaining of chest pain, cough, and joint pain. She has a history of pulmonary sarcoidosis. She states that she has been missing a lot of work because she has been so sick with a variety of complaints.

On physical exam, she weighs 174 pounds. Temp is 98.2. Pulse is 60. Respiratory rate is 24. Blood pressure is 132/90. Lungs: She has coarse breath sounds. Pharynx is slightly erythematous without exudates. Nasal mucosa is pink and moist. Neck is supple with some shotty anterior cervical lymphadenopathy. Heart has a regular rate and rhythm. S1 and S2 without murmur, gallop, or rub. Joints are non-tender, non-erythematous, and have full range of motion with no effusion.

**Studies:** CMP and UA came back normal. Chest x-ray PA and lateral reveals bronchitis and known granulomas of the left lower lobe. EKG was normal.

**Assessment:**
Acute bronchitis
Sarcoidosis
Arthralgias
Elevated blood pressure, not on hypertensive medication

**Plan:** Clarithyromycin 500 mg once a day for 10 days along with Robitussin AC cough syrup 1 teaspoon every 4 hours prn for cough. She will follow-up with her primary care physician next week for her blood pressure which is elevated today. This may be a transient finding due to her breathing issues. Assign the correct **diagnostic** code(s).

Code(s): _____

**1.268.** The following documentation is the discharge progress note from an observation case.

**Nephrology Attending**

Patient is doing somewhat better. Slight cough. Afebrile. Pulmonology has been here to consult. Ordered PEP valve training for airway clearance.

Temp 37, P 115, R22, BP 100/68
No acute distress. Cushingoid facies. RRR with no murmur. Lungs clear bilaterally. Abdomen soft, non-tender, not distended. No edema and no rash.

Blood culture was negative × 24 hours. CXR – mild peribronchial thickening. Urine not sent for culture.

**Assessment/Plan:** Viral URI and neutropenia in a six year old male with Wegener's granulomatosis.

Urine for culture. Respiratory therapy training today. Discharge home after training and ceftriaxone dose this evening. CBC with diff on Monday in my office. Assign the correct **diagnostic** code(s).

Code(s): _____

**1.269.** The patient is a 22-year-old male who had bilateral nasolacrimal duct serial probing with silicone stent placement, completed in the outpatient surgery suite. Assign the correct **diagnostic** code(s).

**Pre- and Postoperative Diagnosis:**
1. Lacrimal duct stenosis, left greater than right
2. Microcephaly
3. Angelman microcephaly syndrome

Code(s): _____

---

**Coding Guideline IV.K. Patients Receiving Diagnostic Services Only**

For patients receiving diagnostic services only during an encounter/visit, sequence first the diagnosis, condition, problem, or other reason for encounter/visit shown in the medical record to be chiefly responsible for the outpatient services provided during the encounter/visit. Codes for other diagnoses (e.g., chronic conditions) may be sequenced as additional diagnoses.

For outpatient encounters for diagnostic tests that have been interpreted by a physician, and the final report is available at the time of coding, code any confirmed or definitive diagnosis(es) documented in the interpretation. Do not code related signs and symptoms as additional diagnoses.

---

**1.270.** The following information is documented on the electrocardiogram report interpreted by the physician:

**Clinical History:** Irregular heart beat

**Findings:** Normal sinus rhythm, bigeminy with frequent PVCs.

Assign the correct **diagnostic** code.

Code(s): _____

**1.271.** The following documentation is from the health record of a male patient who received emergency department services at the community hospital.

**Emergency Department Report**
**Chief Complaint:** Vomiting and stomach ache

**HPI:** 21 month old male with emesis ×4 days. Hard to console today, crying constantly. Vomited at least 3 times for the last four days. Non-bloody, non-bilious vomiting. Today, 1 loose stool. Positive hard stomach with audible bowel sounds last night. Three wet diapers today and positive tears today. Decreased appetite. No fever. No sick contacts. No allergies. No current meds. Immunizations up to date.

**Exam:** General: Screaming during exam. Emesis during exam and not consolable. Head: Fontanel closed. Eyes: Positive tears. ENT: Ears clear, patent tubes bilaterally. Positive rhinorrhea. Moist mucous membranes but lips are dry. Neck: Supple. Chest: Clear to auscultation bilaterally. Tachycardia without murmur. Abdomen: Hard, no audible bowel sounds appreciated. Screaming inconsolably during abdomen exam. GU: Testes high but descended. Lymph nodes: No adenopathy. Skin: Dry with petechiae lower back.

KUB highly suggestive for intussusception. Will bolus fluids and arrange immediate transfer to Children's Hospital for surgical consult and treatment.

**Diagnosis:** Intussusception, acute gastroenteritis, excessive crying, abdominal pain. Assign the correct **diagnostic** code(s).

Code(s): _____

**1.272.** The patient had dental extractions and restoration procedures under general anesthesia as an outpatient. The patient is a child with a history of liver transplant, developmental delay, and dental caries in four deciduous teeth that required extraction and two deciduous teeth that required crowns until permanent teeth develop. Assign the correct **diagnostic** code(s).

**Pre- and Postoperative Diagnosis:**
1. Dental caries, deciduous teeth
2. Global developmental delay
3. Status post liver transplant

Code(s): _____

# ICD-10-CM Coder Training Manual Answer Key

# Introduction to ICD-10-CM Overview

**Activity – New Features in ICD-10-CM**

1. False

2. True

3. By trimester

4. 7

5. 21

## Section 1 Review Questions

1.     c. Musculoskeletal system and connective tissue

2.     a. True

3.     c. Diseases and conditions of the eyes and ears are classified in the same chapter as diseases of the nervous system

4.     b. False

5.     d. All of the above

6.     a. All codes in ICD-10-CM include full code titles

7.     d. N

8.     b. The first character is always an alpha.

9.     b. L03.313

10.     b. False

## Section 2 Review Questions

1.     b. To preserve the meaning of the sixth character

2.     c. NEC

3.     a. True

4.     b. Bracket

5.     b. False

6.     a. True

7.     c. Code first underlying disease

8.     b. The abbreviation NEC

9.     b. False

10.     a. True

## Sections 3 and 4 Review Questions

1.      a. True

2.      b. H10.33

3.      b. False

4.      c. E28.310

5.      b. False

6.      b. False

7.      a. Intractable or not intractable

8.      a. True

9.      a. Dominant

10.     b. The pain code

## Sections 5 and 6 Review Questions

1.      a. True

2.      a. Chapter 13

3.      b. False

4.      b. False

5.      d. Cardiac arrest includes cardiogenic shock

6.      b. False

7.      c. K50.011, K50.014

8.      a. True

9.      a. Septic myocarditis

10.     b. Depth of the ulcer

## Sections 7 and 8 Review Questions

1.      a. True

2.      b. False

3.      c. Eclampsia in the first trimester

4.      b. R10.0

5.      a. A placeholder

6.      a. True

7.      d. P35-P39, Infections specific to the perinatal period

8.      b. False

9.      c. Assigned with the condition discovered coded secondary

10.     a. True

# Final Review Questions

1.      c. October 1, 2014

2.      d. Codes for intraoperative complications and postprocedural disorders have been combined

3.      b. False

4.      b. Note placement

5.      c. As filler so a seventh character may be assigned

6.      b. A diagnosis with an associated sign or symptom

7.      d. Poisoning by medicaments and biological substances

8.      c. N30.11, B96.20

9.      b. Asthmatic bronchitis

10.     d. H65.191

11.     b. M48.46XG

12.     b. False

13.     a. Dominant side

14.     d. All of the above

15.     a. Bilateral cleft palate

16.     a. True

17.     a. Gender

18.     a. First two characters

19.     a. True

20.     c. I21, I22

# ICD-10-CM Coding Conventions and Coding Guidelines Review

## ICD-10-CM Coding Conventions

1.     c. T75.4XXA

2.     c. parentheses

3.     a. True

4.     b. Always a letter

5.     c. *Excludes1*

6.     b. When the information in the medical record provides detail for which a specific code does not exist

7.     a. True

8.     b. False

9.     b. False

10.    b. False

## ICD-10-CM Coding Guidelines

11.    b. The appropriate Z51 code

12.    b. False

13.    a. Liver metastasis

14.    a. True

15.    b. False

16.    b. I21.29, STEMI of other sites; I25.2, Old Myocardial Infarction

17.    c. Highest-degree burn

18.    a. True

19.    d. All of the above

20.    a. True

21.    a. True

22.    c. Congestive heart failure due to hypertension

23.    a. For the trimester in which the complication developed

24.    b. False

25.    a. True

26.     a. True

27.     b. Z21, Asymptomatic HIV infection status

28.     a. Confer with the physician and ask if the condition should be listed as a final diagnosis

29.     b. False

30.     a. A, Initial encounter

# Part I: ICD-10-CM Diagnostic Coding

## Chapter 1 Coding Cases

**1.1.** N39.0    Infection, infected, infective (opportunistic), urinary (tract)

B96.20    Infection, infected, infective (opportunistic), bacterial NOS, as cause of disease classified elsewhere, Escherichia coli [E. coli] (*see also* Escherichia coli)

**1.2.** A04.7    Colitis (acute) (catarrhal) (chronic) (noninfective) (hemorrhagic), Clostridium difficile

Z16.39    Resistance, resistant (to), organism(s), to, drug, antimicrobial (single), specified NEC

**1.3.** M62.561    Atrophy, atrophic (of), muscle, muscular (diffuse) (general) Idiopathic) (primary), lower leg

B91    Late effect(s) – *see* Sequelae, Sequelae (of), poliomyelitis (acute)

**1.4.** A02.9    Poisoning (acute), food (acute) (diseased) (infected) (noxious), bacterial – *see* Intoxication, foodborne, by agent, Intoxication, foodborne, due to Salmonella

**1.5.** A56.11    Disease, diseased, sexually transmitted, chlamydial infection – *see* Chlamydia, female, pelvic inflammatory disease

**1.6.** B20    AIDS (related complex)

B59    Pneumonia, Pneumocystis (carinii) (jiroveci)

**1.7.** A41.51    Sepsis (generalized), Escherichia coli (E. Coli). Review Tabular for complete code assignment.

**1.8.** A41.50    Sepsis (generalized), gram-negative (organism). Review Tabular for complete code assignment.

R65.20    Sepsis, with, organ dysfunction (acute) (multiple)

J96.00    Failure, failed, respiration, respiratory, acute

**1.9.** A39.2    Sepsis (generalized), meningococcal, acute

R65.21    Shock, septic (due to severe sepsis)

**1.10.** N20.0    Nephrolithiasis (congenital) (pelvis) (recurrent) - *see also* Calculus, kidney, Calculus, calculi, calculous, kidney (impacted) (multiple) (pelvis) (recurrent) (staghorn)

J15.1    Pneumonia, Pseudomonas, NEC

Y95    Index to External Causes, Nosocomial condition

**1.11.** B18.1    Hepatitis, viral, virus, chronic, type B

## Chapter 2 Coding Cases

**1.12.**  C34.31     Carcinoma, *see also* Neoplasm, by site, malignant. Refer to Neoplasm Table, by site (lung), malignant, primary site, lower lobe.

    C77.1      Refer to Neoplasm Table, by site, lymph gland, malignant, intrathoracic, secondary site.

    C79.31     Refer to Neoplasm Table, by site, brain, malignant, secondary site.

    C79.51     Refer to Neoplasm Table, by site, bone, malignant, rib, secondary site.

**1.13.**  D3A.021    Carcinoid, *see* Tumor, carcinoid, benign, cecum

**1.14.**  C93.91     Leukemia, leukemic, monocytic (subacute)

**1.15.**  C43.52     Melanoma (malignant), skin, breast (female) (male)

    C43.62     Melanoma (malignant), skin, arm. Review the Tabular for complete code assignment.

**1.16.**  E86.0      Dehydration

    G89.3      Pain(s) (*see also* Painful), chronic, neoplasm related

    C50.111    Carcinoma, *see also* Neoplasm, by site, malignant. Refer to Neoplasm Table, by site (breast), malignant, primary site, central portion.

    C79.31     Refer to Neoplasm Table, by site, brain, malignant, secondary site.

    C78.7      Refer to Neoplasm Table, by site, liver, malignant, secondary site.

**1.17.**  C79.31     Refer to Neoplasm Table, by site, brain, malignant, secondary site

    Z85.3      History, personal (of), malignant neoplasm (of), breast

    Z90.12     Absence (of) (organ or part) (complete or partial), breast(s) (and nipple(s)) (acquired)

    Z92.21     History, personal (of), chemotherapy for neoplastic condition

**1.18.**  Z51.11     Chemotherapy (session) (for), cancer

    C17.8      Carcinoma, *see also* Neoplasm, by site, malignant. Refer to Neoplasm Table, by site, intestine, small, overlapping lesion, malignant, primary site.

    Z90.49     Absence (of) (organ or part) (complete or partial), intestine (acquired) (small)

## Chapter 3 Coding Cases

**1.19.**  C50.912    Carcinoma, *see also* Neoplasm, by site, malignant. Neoplasm, breast (connective tissue) (glandular tissue) (soft parts)

    D63.0      Anemia (essential) (general) (hemoglobin deficiency) (infantile) (primary) (profound), in (due to) (with), neoplastic disease (*see also* Neoplasm)

**1.20.**  D61.01     Anemia (essential) (general) (hemoglobin deficiency) (infantile) (primary) (profound), aplastic, red cell (pure), congenital

**1.21.**  D70.4      Neutropenia, neutropenic (chronic) (genetic) (idiopathic) (immune) (infantile) (malignant) (pernicious) (splenic), periodic

**1.22.**  D56.3      Thalassemia (anemia) (disease), minor

**1.23.**  D57.01     Anemia, sickle-cell – *see* Disease, sickle-cell, with crisis (vasoocclusive pain), with, acute chest syndrome

**1.24.**  D81.1      Immunodeficiency, combined, severe (SCID), with, low T- and B-cell numbers

## Chapter 4 Coding Cases

**1.25.** E11.321     Diabetes, diabetic (mellitus) (sugar), type 2, with, retinopathy, nonproliferative, mild, with macular edema

       E11.36      Diabetes, diabetic (mellitus) (sugar), type 2, with, cataract

       Z79.4       Long-term (current) (prophylactic) drug therapy (use of), insulin

**1.26.** E10.22      Diabetes, diabetic (mellitus) (sugar) type 1, with, chronic kidney disease

       N18.3       Disease, diseased, kidney (functional) (pelvis), chronic, stage 3 (moderate)

       K04.7       Abscess, tooth, teeth (root)

**1.27.** K85.0       Pancreatitis (annular) (apoplectic) (calcareous) (edematous) (hemorrhagic) (malignant) (recurrent) (subacute) (suppurative), acute, idiopathic

       E08.65      Diabetes, diabetic (mellitus) (sugar), due to underlying condition, with, hyperglycemia

       Z79.4       Long-term (current) (prophylactic) drug therapy (use of), insulin

**1.28.** E66.01      Obesity, morbid

       Z68.41      Body, bodies, mass index (BMI), adult, 40.0–44.9

**1.29.** F50.2       Bulimia (nervosa)

       E44.0       Malnutrition, protein, calorie, moderate

**1.30.** E86.0       Dehydration

       A02.0       Gastroenteritis (acute) (chronic) (noninfectious), Salmonella or Infection, Salmonella, with (gastro)enteritis

**1.31.** E10.10      Diabetes, diabetic (mellitus) (sugar), type 1, with, ketoacidosis

       E86.0       Dehydration

**1.32.** E09.9       Diabetes, diabetic, (mellitus) (sugar) due to drug or chemical

       T38.0X5S   Refer to Table of Drugs and Chemicals, Corticosteroid, adverse effect

       Z79.4       Long-term (current) (prophylactic) drug therapy (use of), insulin

**1.33.** E05.20      Hyperthyroidism (latent) (pre-adult) (recurrent) with, goiter (diffuse), nodular (multinodular)

       R00.2       Palpitations (heart)

**1.34.** E10.621     Diabetes, diabetic (mellitus) (sugar), type 1, with foot ulcer

       L97.521     Ulcer, foot, *see* Ulcer, lower limb, lower limb, foot, left, with skin breakdown only

       E10.51      Diabetes, diabetic (mellitus) (sugar), type 1, with peripheral angiopathy

       E10.22      Diabetes, diabetic (mellitus) (sugar), type 1, with chronic kidney disease

       N18.2       Disease, diseased, kidney (functional) (pelvis), chronic, stage 2 (mild)

## Chapter 5 Coding Cases

**1.35.** F10.129     Abuse, alcohol (non-dependent), with, intoxication

**1.36.** F15.20      Dependence (on) (syndrome), amphetamine(s) (type), *see* Dependence, drug, stimulant, NEC

**1.37.** Z71.6      Counseling (for), tobacco use
          F17.220    Dependence, (on) (syndrome), nicotine, *see* Dependence, drug, nicotine. Dependence, drug, nicotine, chewing tobacco

**1.38.** F10.20    Dependence, (on) (syndrome), alcohol (ethyl) (methyl) (without remission)
          K29.20    Gastritis (simple), alcoholic
          F14.21    History, personal (of), drug dependence – *see* Dependence, drug, by type, in remission. Dependence, (on) (syndrome), drug, cocaine, in remission

**1.39.** F60.3      Disorder, personality, borderline
          F10.21    Alcohol, alcoholic, alcohol-induced, addiction, with remission
          Z79.899   Long-term (current) (prophylactic) drug therapy (use of), drug, specified NEC

**1.40.** F10.229   Intoxication, alcoholic (acute) (without dependence) –*see* Alcohol, intoxication. Alcohol, alcoholic, alcohol-induced, intoxication (acute) (without dependence), with, dependence
          Y90.1     Index to External Causes, Blood alcohol level, 20–39mg/100ml

## *Chapter 6 Coding Cases*

**1.41.** G30.0      Alzheimer's disease or sclerosis, *see* Disease, Alzheimer's, early onset, with behavioral disturbance
          F02.81    Dementia, in Alzheimer's disease, *see* Disease, Alzheimer's
          Z91.83    Wandering, in diseases classified elsewhere

**1.42.** G40.B19   Epilepsy, epileptic, epilepsia (attack) (cerebral) (convulsion) (fit) (seizure), juvenile myoclonic, intractable

**1.43.** G81.94    Hemiplegia. Review Tabular for complete code assignment.

**1.44.** G00.1      Meningitis, pneumococcal
          J13        Pneumonia, pneumococcal, (broncho) (lobar)

**1.45.** G21.11    Parkinsonism (idiopathic) (primary), secondary, due to drugs, neuroleptic
          T43.4X5A   Refer to Table of Drugs and Chemicals, Haloperidol, adverse effect
          F20.0     Schizophrenia, paranoid (type)

**1.46.** G89.3      Pain(s) (*see also* Painful), acute, neoplasm related
          C50.911   Refer to Neoplasm Table, by site, breast, malignant, primary site.
          C78.7     Refer to Neoplasm Table, by site, liver, malignant, secondary site.

**1.47.** G45.9      Attack, attacks, transient ischemic (TIA)
          E11.40    Diabetes, diabetic, (mellitus) (sugar) type 2, with, neuropathy
          G43.119   Migraine, classical – *see* Migraine, with aura. Migraine, with aura, intractable

## *Chapter 7 Coding Cases*

**1.48.** H01.001   Blepharitis (angularis) (ciliaris) (eyelid) (marginal) (nonulcerative), right, upper
          H01.004   Blepharitis (angularis) (ciliaris) (eyelid) (marginal) (nonulcerative), left, upper

**1.49.**  H11.063       Pterygium (eye), recurrent. See Tabular for correct code assignment.

**1.50.**  H25.12        Cataract (cortical) (immature) (incipient), age-related – *see* Cataract, senile, nuclear (sclerosis)

**1.51.**  H40.11X2      Glaucoma, open angle, primary. See Tabular for complete code assignment.

**1.52.**  H59.012       Keratopathy, bullous (aphakic), following cataract surgery

**1.53.**  H25.011       Cataract (cortical) (immature) (incipient), age-related, *see* Cataract, senile, cortical

   H59.311       Hemorrhage, postoperative, *see* Complications, postprocedural, hemorrhage, by site
               Complication(s) (from) (of), postprocedural, hemorrhage (hematoma) (of), eye and adnexa, following ophthalmic procedure

   Y92.530       Index to External Causes, Place of occurrence, outpatient surgery center

## Chapter 8 Coding Cases

**1.54.**  H65.02        Otitis (acute), media (hemorrhagic) (staphylococcal) (streptococcal) acute, subacute, serous – *see* Otitis, media, nonsuppurative, acute, serous. Otitis media, nonsuppurative, acute or subacute, serous

   H66.91        Otitis (acute), media (hemorrhagic) (staphylococcal) (streptococcal), chronic

   H72.821       Perforation, perforated (nontraumatic) (of), tympanum, tympanic (membrane) (persistent post-traumatic) (postinflammatory), total

**1.55.**  H81.02        Vertigo, Ménière's – *see* subcategory H81.0

**1.56.**  H80.03        Otosclerosis (general) involving oval window, nonobliterative

   H90.0         Loss (of), hearing – *see* also Deafness. Deafness, conductive, bilateral

   H95.31        Complication(s), ear procedure, laceration – *see* Complications, intraoperative, puncture or laceration, ear. Complication(s) intraoperative, puncture or laceration (accidental) (unintentional) (of) ear, during procedure on ear and mastoid process

   Y92.234       Index to External Causes, Place of occurrence, hospital, operating room

## Chapter 9 Coding Cases

**1.57.**  I10           Hypertension, hypertensive, (accelerated) (benign) (essential) (idiopathic) (malignant) (systemic)

**1.58.**  I13.0         Hypertension, hypertensive, (accelerated) (benign) (essential) (idiopathic) (malignant) (systemic), cardiorenal (disease), with heart failure, with stage 1 through stage 4 chronic kidney disease

   I50.9         Failure, failed, heart (acute) (senile) (sudden), congestive (compensated) (decompensated)

   N18.3         Disease, diseased, kidney (functional) (pelvis), chronic, stage 3 (moderate)

**1.59.**  I21.4         Infarct, Infarction, myocardium, myocardial (acute) (with stated duration of 4 weeks or less), non-ST elevation (NSTEMI)

   I48.91        Fibrillation, atrial or auricular (established)

**1.60.**  I22.1    Infarct, Infarction, myocardium, myocardial (acute) (with stated duration of 4 weeks or less), subsequent (recurrent) (reinfarction), inferior (diaphragmatic) (inferolateral) (inferoposterior) (wall)

  I21.4    Infarct, Infarction, myocardium, myocardial (acute) (with stated duration of 4 weeks or less), non-ST elevation (NSTEMI)

  I48.91   Fibrillation, atrial or auricular (established)

**1.61.**  I23.7    Angina (attack) (cardiac) (chest) (heart) (pectoris) (syndrome) (vasomotor), post-infarctional

  I21.09   Infarct, infarction, myocardium, myocardial (acute) (with stated duration of 4 weeks or less), ST elevation (STEMI), anterior (anteroapical) (anterolateral) (anteroseptal) (Q wave) (wall)

**1.62.**  I25.119  Disease, diseased, coronary (artery) – *see* Disease, heart, ischemic, atherosclerotic (of), with angina pectoris – *see* Arteriosclerosis, coronary (artery), native vessel, with angina pectoris

**1.63.**  I25.110  Angina (attack) (cardiac) (chest) (heart) (pectoris) (syndrome) (vasomotor), with atherosclerotic heart disease – *see* Arteriosclerosis, coronary (artery), native vessel with angina pectoris, unstable

  I69.351  Hemiparesis – *see* Hemiplegia, following, cerebrovascular disease, cerebral infarction

  Z95.1    Status (post), aortocoronary bypass

**1.64.**  I50.33   Failure, failed, heart (acute) (senile) (sudden), diastolic (congestive), acute (congestive), and (on) chronic (congestive)

**1.65.**  I63.322  Infarct, infarction, cerebral – (*see also* Occlusion, artery, cerebral or precerebral, with infarction). Occlusion, artery, cerebral, anterior, with infarction, due to, thrombosis. or Infarct, infarction, cerebral, due to thrombosis, cerebral artery. Review the Tabular for correct code assignment.

  G81.91   Hemiplegia. Review the Tabular for correct code assignment.

**1.66.**  I69.354  Hemiparesis – *see* Hemiplegia, following, cerebrovascular disease, stroke

  I69.320  Aphasia, following cerebrovascular disease, cerebral infarction

**1.67.**  I25.110  Angina (attack) (cardiac) (chest) (heart) (pectoris) (syndrome) (vasomotor), with atherosclerotic heart disease – *see* Arteriosclerosis, coronary (artery), native vessel with angina pectoris, unstable

  I25.2    Infarct, infarction, myocardium, myocardial, healed or old

**1.68.**  I25.720  Atherosclerosis – *see also* Arteriosclerosis, coronary artery, with angina pectoris, – *see* Arteriosclerosis, coronary (artery), bypass graft, autologous artery, with, angina pectoris, unstable

  I11.0    Failure, failed, heart (acute) (senile) (sudden), hypertensive – *see* Hypertension, heart (disease) (conditions in I51.4-I51.9 due to hypertension), with, heart failure (congestive)

  I50.9    Failure, failed, heart (acute) (senile) (sudden), congestive (compensated)

**1.69.**  I21.19   Infarct, infarction, myocardium, myocardial (acute) (with stated duration of 4 weeks or less), ST elevation (STEMI), inferior (diaphragmatic) (inferolateral) (inferoposterior) (wall), NEC

  I23.0    Hemopericardium, following acute myocardial infarction (current complication)

**1.70.** I63.442  Infarct, infarction, cerebellar – *see* Infarct, cerebral. (*See also* Occlusion, artery, cerebral or precerebral, with infarction.) Occlusion, occluded artery, cerebellar (anterior inferior) (posterior inferior) (superior) with infarction, due to, embolism. Review the Tabular for complete and correct code assignment.

R13.10  Dysphagia

G81.91  Hemiplegia. Review the Tabular for complete code assignment.

## Chapter 10 Coding Cases

**1.71.** J14  Pneumonia (acute) (double) (migratory) (purulent) (septic) (unresolved), Hemophilus influenza (broncho) (lobar)

**1.72.** J44.1  Disease, diseased, pulmonary, chronic obstructive, with exacerbation (acute)

F17.200  Dependence (on) (syndrome), tobacco – *see* Dependence, drug, nicotine

Z71.6  Counseling (for), substance abuse, tobacco

**1.73.** J45.51  Asthma, asthmatic (bronchial) (catarrh) (spasmodic), persistent, severe, with exacerbation (acute)

**1.74.** J96.00  Failure, respiration, respiratory, acute

J44.0  Bronchitis (diffuse) (fibrinous) (hypostatic) (infective) (membranous), acute or subacute, with chronic obstructive pulmonary disease

J20.9  Bronchitis (diffuse) (fibrinous) (hypostatic) (infective) (membranous), acute or subacute

J44.1  Disease, diseased, pulmonary, chronic obstructive, with exacerbation (acute)

**1.75.** J69.0  Pneumonia, aspiration, due to food (regurgitated)

K21.9  Reflux, gastroesophageal

**1.76.** J09.X2  Influenza (bronchial) (epidemic) (respiratory) (upper) (unidentified influenza virus), due to identified novel influenza A virus, with, respiratory manifestations, NEC

**1.77.** J43.9  Emphysema (atrophic) (bullous) (chronic) (interlobular) (lung) (obstructive) (pulmonary) (senile) (vesicular)

I50.9  Failure, failed, heart (acute) (senile) (sudden), congestive (compensated) (decompensated)

I10  Hypertension, hypertensive (accelerated) (benign) (essential) (idiopathic) (malignant) (systemic)

I48.91  Fibrillation, atrial or auricular (established)

**1.78.** J45.42  Asthma, asthmatic, moderate persistent, with, status asthmaticus

J44.1  Disease, lung, obstructive (chronic), with, acute, exacerbation NEC

**1.79.** E86.0  Dehydration

J43.9  Emphysema (atrophic) (bullous) (chronic) (interlobular) (lung) (obstructive) (pulmonary) (senile) (vesicular)

Z99.11  Dependence, on, ventilator

**1.80.** J69.0     Pneumonia, aspiration, due to food (regurgitated)

I69.391     Dysphagia, following, cerebrovascular disease, cerebral infarction

R13.19     Dysphagia, neurogenic

L89.211     Ulcer, decubitus – *see* Ulcer, pressure by site

         Ulcer, pressure, stage 1 (healing) (pre-ulcer skin changes limited to persistent focal edema), hip, right

L89.221     Ulcer, pressure, Ulcer, pressure, stage 1 (healing) (pre-ulcer skin changes limited to persistent focal edema), hip, left

## Chapter 11 Coding Cases

**1.81.** K40.41     Hernia, hernial, (acquired) (recurrent), inguinal (direct) (external) (funicular) (indirect) (internal) (oblique) (scrotal) (sliding), unilateral, with, gangrene (and obstruction), recurrent

**1.82.** K25.0     Ulcer, ulcerated, ulcerating, ulceration, ulcerative, gastric – *see* Ulcer, stomach (eroded) (peptic) (round), acute, with, hemorrhage

**1.83.** K80.33     Choledocholithiasis (common duct) (hepatic duct) – *see* Calculus, bile duct (common) (hepatic), with, cholangitis, acute, with, obstruction

**1.84.** K50.012     Crohn's disease – *see* Enteritis, regional, Enteritis (acute) (diarrheal) (hemorrhagic) (noninfective) (septic), regional (of), small intestine, with complication, intestinal obstruction

**1.85.** K25.4     Ulcer, ulcerated, ulcerating, ulceration, ulcerative, gastric – *see* ulcer, stomach (eroded) (peptic) (round), chronic, with hemorrhage

I50.9     Failure, failed, heart (acute) (senile) (sudden), congestive (compensated) (decompensated)

I48.91     Fibrillation, atrial or auricular (established)

**1.86.** K40.20     Hernia, hernial (acquired) (recurrent), inguinal (direct) (external) (funicular) (indirect) (internal) (oblique) (scrotal) (sliding), bilateral

R07.2     Pain(s) (*see also* Painful), chest (central), precordial

J44.9     Disease, diseased, pulmonary, chronic obstructive

M54.5     Pain(s) (*see also* Painful), low back

I10     Hypertension, hypertensive (accelerated) (benign) (essential) (idiopathic) (malignant) (systemic)

Z53.09     Canceled procedure (surgical), because of contraindication

**1.87.** K94.22     Complication(s) (from) (of), gastrostomy (stoma), infection

L03.311     Cellulitis (diffuse) (phlegmonous) (septic) (suppurative), abdominal wall

C15.4     Neoplasm Table, by site (esophagus), malignant, primary

B95.62     Infection, infected, infective (opportunistic), staphylococcal, as cause of disease classified elsewhere, aureus, methicillin resistant

## *Chapter 12 Coding Cases*

**1.88.** L27.0 — Dermatitis (eczematous), due to, drugs and medicaments (generalized) (internal use)

T36.0X5A — Table of Drugs and Chemicals, Penicillin (any), Adverse Effect, initial encounter

**1.89.** I96 — Ulcer, gangrenous – *see* Gangrene. Gangrene, gangrenous (connective tissue) (dropsical) (dry) (moist) (skin) (ulcer) (*see also* necrosis). Necrosis, skin or subcutaneous tissue NEC

L89.213 — Ulcer, ulcerated, ulcerating, ulceration, ulcerative, pressure (pressure area) stage 3, (healing) (full thickness skin loss involving damage or necrosis of subcutaneous tissue), hip. Review the Tabular for complete code assignment.

L89.152 — Ulcer, ulcerated, ulcerating, ulceration, ulcerative, pressure (pressure area) stage 2, (healing) (abrasion, blister, partial thickness skin loss involving epidermis and/or dermis) sacral region (tailbone). Review the Tabular for complete code assignment.

L03.115 — Cellulitis (diffuse) (phlegmonous) (septic) (suppurative), hip – *see* Cellulitis, lower limb. Review the Tabular for complete code assignment.

**1.90.** I70.233 — Atherosclerosis, *see also* arteriosclerosis. Arteriosclerosis, arteriosclerotic (diffuse) (obliterans) (of) (senile) (with calcification), extremities (native arteries) leg, right, with ulceration (and intermittent claudication and rest pain), ankle

L97.311 — Ulcer, ulcerated, ulcerating, ulceration, ulcerative, lower limb (atrophic) (chronic) (neurogenic) (perforating) (pyogenic) (trophic) (tropical) ankle, right, with skin breakdown only

**1.91.** L02.612 — Abscess (connective tissue) (embolic) (fistulous) (infective) (metastatic) (multiple) (pernicious) (pyogenic) (septic), toe (any) *see also* Abscess, foot. Abscess, foot

I96 — Gangrene, gangrenous (connective tissue) (dropsical) (dry) (moist) (skin) (ulcer) (*see also* necrosis). Necrosis, skin or subcutaneous tissue NEC

**1.92.** L03.115 — Cellulitis, leg – *see* Cellulitis, lower limb. Lower limb

B95.1 — Infection, bacterial NOS, as cause of disease classified elsewhere, Streptococcus group B

L89.312 — Ulcer, ulcerated, ulcerating, ulceration, ulcerative, decubitus – *see* Ulcer, pressure, by site. Pressure (pressure area) stage 2, (healing) (abrasion, blister, partial thickness skin loss involving epidermis and/or dermis), buttock

L89.321 — Ulcer, ulcerated, ulcerating, ulceration, ulcerative, decubitus – *see* Ulcer, pressure, by site. Pressure (pressure area) stage 1, (healing) (pre-ulcer skin changes limited to persistent focal edema), buttock

**1.93.** L27.1 — Dermatitis, (eczematous) due to drugs and medicaments, (generalized) (internal use) localized skin eruption

T46.4X5A — Table of Drugs and Chemicals, Ramipril, Adverse Effect, initial encounter

I10 — Hypertension, hypertensive (accelerated) (benign) (essential) (idiopathic) (malignant) (systemic)

**1.94.** L24.3      Dermatitis (eczematous), contact, irritant, due to, cosmetics
        H01.114      Dermatitis (eczematous), eyelid, contact – *see* Dermatitis, eyelid, allergic, left, upper
        H01.111      Dermatitis (eczematous), eyelid, contact – *see* Dermatitis, eyelid, allergic, right, upper
        T49.8X5A      Table of Drugs and Chemicals, Cosmetics, adverse effect
        L70.0      Acne, cystic

**1.95.** L03.221      Cellulitis (diffuse) (phlegmonous) (septic) (suppurative), neck (region)
        F11.10      Abuse, drug, morphine type (opioids) – *see* Abuse, drug, opioid. Opioid
        Z72.89      Behavior, drug seeking

## *Chapter 13 Coding Cases*

**1.96.** M00.861      Arthritis, arthritic (acute) (chronic) (nonpyogenic) (subacute), septic (any site except spine) – *see* Arthritis, pyogenic or pyemic (any site except spine), bacterial NEC, knee. Review the Tabular for correct code assignment.

**1.97.** M08.071      Arthritis, arthritic (acute) (chronic) (nonpyogenic) (subacute), rheumatoid, juvenile (with or without rheumatoid factor), ankle. Review the Tabular for assignment of laterality.
        M08.072      Arthritis, arthritic (acute) (chronic) (nonpyogenic) (subacute), rheumatoid, juvenile (with or without rheumatoid factor), ankle. Review the Tabular for assignment of laterality.

**1.98.** M84.551A      Fracture, pathological (pathologic), due to neoplastic disease, femur
        C79.51      Carcinoma (malignant), metastatic, *see* Neoplasm, secondary. Refer to Neoplasm Table, by site, bone, femur, secondary.
        Z85.118      History, personal (of), malignant neoplasm (of), lung
        Z92.3      History, personal (of), radiation therapy

**1.99.** M80.08XA      Fracture, pathological (pathologic), due to osteoporosis, specified cause NEC – *see* Osteoporosis, specified type NEC, with pathological fracture. Osteoporosis (female) (male), senile – *see* Osteoporosis, age-related, with current pathologic fracture, vertebra(e)

## *Chapter 14 Coding Cases*

**1.100.** N03.2      Syndrome, nephritic – *see also* Nephritis. Nephritis, nephritic, chronic, with diffuse membranous glomerulonephritis.

**1.101.** N30.01      Cystitis (exudative) (hemorrhagic) (septic) (suppurative), acute, with hematuria
        B96.20      Escherichia (E.) coli, as cause of disease classified elsewhere

**1.102.** N92.4      Menorrhagia (primary), preclimacteric or premenopausal

**1.103.** N17.0     Failure, failed, kidney, acute (*see also* Failure, renal, acute). Failure, renal, acute, with, tubular necrosis

       N40.1     Hypertrophy, prostate – *see* Enlargement, enlarged, prostate, with lower urinary tract symptoms (LUTS)

       N13.8     Obstruction, urinary (moderate)

**1.104.** N18.3     Disease, diseased, kidney (functional) (pelvis), chronic, stage 3 (moderate)

       Z94.0     Status (post), transplant – *see* Transplant, kidney

       E89.0     Hypothyroidism (acquired), postsurgical

       Z85.850     History, personal (of), malignant neoplasm (of), thyroid

**1.105.** N39.0     Infection, infected, infective, (opportunistic), urinary (tract)

       B96.4     Infection, infected, infective (opportunistic), bacterial NOS, as cause of disease classified elsewhere, proteus (mirabilis) (morganii)

       Z87.440     History, personal (of), infection, urinary (recurrent) (tract)

## *Chapter 15 Coding Cases*

**1.106.** O13.2     Pregnancy (single) (uterine) , complicated by (care of) (management affected by), hypertension, – *see* Hypertension, complicating, pregnancy, gestational (pregnancy induced) (transient) (without proteinuria). Review the Tabular for complete code assignment.

       O09.522     Pregnancy (single) (uterine) , complicated by (care of) (management affected by), elderly, multigravida. Review the Tabular for complete code assignment.

       Z3A.26     Pregnancy (single) (uterine), weeks of gestation, 26 weeks

**1.107.** O21.0     Pregnancy (single) (uterine) , complicated by (care of) (management affected by), hyperemesis (gravidarum) (mild) – *see also* Hyperemesis, gravidarum (mild)

       O23.42     Pregnancy (single) (uterine) , complicated by (care of) (management affected by), infection(s), urinary (tract). Review the Tabular for complete code assignment.

       B96.20     Infection, infected, infective (opportunistic), bacterial NOS, as cause of disease classified elsewhere, Escherichia coli [E. coli]

       Z3A.16     Pregnancy (single) (uterine), weeks of gestation, 16 weeks

**1.108.** O91.22     Mastitis (acute) (diffuse) (nonpuerperal) (subacute), obstetric (interstitial) (nonpurulent), associated with, puerperium

**1.109.** O30.003     Pregnancy (single) (uterine) , complicated by (care of) (management affected by), multiple gestations, twin *see* Pregnancy, twin. Review the Tabular for complete code assignment.

       O69.81X2     Delivery (childbirth) (labor), complicated, by, cord (umbilical), around neck, without compression. Review the Tabular for seventh character.

       Z3A.39     Pregnancy (single) (uterine), weeks of gestation, 39 weeks

       Z37.2     Outcome of delivery, twins NEC, both liveborn

**1.110.** O24.419     Pregnancy (single) (uterine) , complicated by (care of) (management affected by), diabetes (mellitus), gestational (pregnancy induced) *see* Diabetes, gestational (in pregnancy)

       Z3A.28     Pregnancy (single) (uterine), weeks of gestation, 28 weeks

**1.111.** O26.12    Pregnancy (single) (uterine) , complicated by (care of) (management affected by), insufficient, weight gain. Review the Tabular for complete code assignment.

        O10.012    Pregnancy (single) (uterine) , complicated by (care of) (management affected by), hypertension, *see* Hypertension, complicating, pregnancy, pre-existing, essential. Review the Tabular for complete code assignment.

        Z3A.20    Pregnancy (single) (uterine), weeks of gestation, 20 weeks

**1.112.** O80    Delivery (childbirth) (labor), normal

        Z3A.39    Pregnancy (single) (uterine), weeks of gestation, 39 weeks

        Z37.0    Outcome of delivery, single, liveborn

**1.113.** O70.1    Delivery (childbirth) (labor), complicated, by, laceration (perineal), perineum, perineal, second degree

        Z3A.38    Pregnancy (single) (uterine), weeks of gestation, 38 weeks

        Z37.0    Outcome of delivery, single, liveborn

**1.114.** O98.712    Pregnancy (single) (uterine) , complicated by (care of ) (management affected by), human immunodeficiency [HIV] disease. Review the Tabular for complete code assignment.

        B20    AIDS (related complex)

        B59    Pneumocystis carinii pneumonia

        Z3A.21    Pregnancy (single) (uterine), weeks of gestation, 21 weeks

**1.115.** O60.14X2    Pregnancy (single) (uterine) , complicated by (care of) (management affected by), preterm labor, third trimester, with third trimester preterm delivery

        O36.4XX2    Pregnancy (single) (uterine) , complicated by (care of ) (management affected by), fetal (maternal care for), death (near term) or Pregnancy, complicated by, intrauterine fetal death (near term). Review the Tabular for complete code assignment.

        O30.103    Pregnancy (single) (uterine) , complicated by (care of ) (management affected by), multiple gestations, triplet, *see* Pregnancy, triplet – *see* Tabular for complete code, triplet

        O41.1030    Pregnancy (single) (uterine), complicated by (care of) (management affected by), infection(s), amniotic fluid or sac

        Z3A.34    Pregnancy (single) (uterine), weeks of gestation, 34 weeks

        Z37.61    Outcome of delivery, multiple births, some liveborn, triplets

**1.116.** O86.0    Complication(s) (from) (of), obstetric, surgical wound NEC, infection; Infection, obstetrical surgical wound (puerperal)

        B95.1    Infection, infected, infective (opportunistic) bacterial, as cause of disease classified elsewhere, Streptococcus, group B

**1.117.** O34.21    Delivery (childbirth) (labor), cesarean (for), previous, cesarean delivery

        O64.3XX0    Delivery (childbirth) (labor), complicated, by, obstructed labor, due to, brow presentation

        O66.41    Delivery (childbirth) (labor), complicated, by, failed, attempted vaginal birth after previous cesarean delivery

        Z3A.39    Pregnancy (single) (uterine), weeks of gestation, 39 weeks

        Z37.0    Outcome of delivery, single, liveborn

**1.118.** O03.4      Abortion (complete) (spontaneous), incomplete (spontaneous)

O13.1      Hypertension, complicating, pregnancy, gestational (pregnancy induced) (transient) (without proteinuria)

Z3A.12      Pregnancy (single) (uterine), weeks of gestation, 12 weeks

## Chapter 16 Coding Cases

**1.119.** P36.2      Newborn, (infant) (liveborn) (singleton), sepsis (congenital), due to Staphylococcus, aureus

**1.120.** P59.9      Newborn (infant) (liveborn) (singleton), hyperbilirubinemia

**1.121.** Z38.00      Newborn (infant) (liveborn) (singleton), born in hospital

Q86.0      Syndrome, fetal, alcohol (dysmorphic)

**1.122.** Z38.01      Newborn (infant) (liveborn) (singleton), born in hospital, by cesarean

P04.41      Newborn (infant) (liveborn) (singleton), affected by cocaine (crack)

P07.14      Weight, 1000–2499 grams at birth (low) – *see* Low, birth weight. Low, birth weight (2499 grams or less) with weight of 1000–1249 grams

P07.34      Premature, newborn, less than 37 completed weeks – *see* Preterm newborn. Preterm, newborn (infant), gestational age 31 completed weeks (31 weeks, 0 days through 31 weeks, 6 days)

P74.1      Newborn (infant) (liveborn) (singleton), dehydration

## Chapter 17 Coding Cases

**1.123.** Q01.0      Encephalocele, frontal

**1.124.** Q37.4      Cleft, (congenital) lip (unilateral), bilateral, with cleft palate, hard with soft

**1.125.** Q54.2      Hypospadias, penoscrotal

**1.126.** Z38.01      Newborn (infant) (liveborn) (singleton), born in hospital, by cesarean

Q20.3      Transposition (congenital) vessels, great (complete) (partial)

## Chapter 18 Coding Cases

**1.127.** R10.821      Tenderness, abdominal, rebound, right upper quadrant

**1.128.** R40.2111      Coma, with opening of eyes (never)

R40.2211      Coma, with verbal response (none)

R40.2311      Coma, with motor response (none)

R40.2134      Coma, with opening of eyes, in response to sound

R40.2234      Coma, with verbal response, inappropriate words

R40.2344      Coma, with motor response, flexion withdrawal

**1.129.** R92.0      Microcalcifications, breast

**1.130.** R00.1      Bradycardia (sinoatrial) (sinus) (vagal)

**1.131.** R07.89      Pain(s) (*see also* Painful), chest (central), atypical

I20.9      Angina (attack) (cardiac) (chest) (heart) (pectoris) (syndrome) (vasomotor)

K21.9      Disease, diseased, gastroesophageal reflux (GERD)

**1.132.** R50.9 Fever (inanition) (of unknown origin) (persistent) (with chills) (with rigor)

**1.133.** R10.11 Pain(s) (*see also* Painful), abdominal, upper, right quadrant
R11.2 Nausea, with vomiting
R03.0 Elevated, elevation, blood pressure, reading (incidental) (isolated) (nonspecific), no diagnosis of hypertension

## *Chapter 19 Coding Cases*

**1.134.** T74.4XXA Syndrome, shaken infant

**1.135.** S82.852K Nonunion, fracture – *see* Fracture, by site. Fracture, traumatic (abduction) (adduction) (separation), ankle, trimalleolar (displaced). Review the Tabular for complete code assignment as well as correct seventh character.

**1.136.** S52.351B Fracture, traumatic (abduction) (adduction) (separation), radius, shaft, comminuted (displaced). Review the Tabular for complete code assignment, including the seventh character.

**1.137.** G82.21 Paraplegia (lower), complete
S32.029S Fracture, traumatic (abduction) (adduction) (separation), vertebra, vertebral (arch) (body) (column) (neural arch) (pedicle) (spinous process) (transverse process), lumbar, second. Review the Tabular for correct seventh character.

**1.138.** S02.65XG Fracture, traumatic, (abduction) (adduction) (separation), mandible (lower jaw (bone)), angle (of jaw). Review the Tabular for complete code assignment and correct seventh character.

**1.139.** S02.0XXA Fracture, traumatic (abduction) (adduction) (separation), skull, frontal bone. Review the Tabular for complete code assignment.
S06.5X2A Hemorrhage, hemorrhagic (concealed), intracranial (nontraumatic), subdural, traumatic – *see* Injury, intracranial (traumatic), subdural hemorrhage, traumatic. Review the Tabular for complete code assignment and correct seventh character.

**1.140.** S91.322A Laceration, heel – *see* Laceration, foot (except toe(s) alone), left, with foreign body. Review the Tabular for correct seventh character.

**1.141.** S42.431D Fracture, traumatic (abduction) (adduction) (separation), humerus, lower end, epicondyle, lateral (displaced). Review the Tabular for complete code assignment and the correct seventh character.

**1.142.** T39.1X1A Poisoning (acute) - *see* also Table of Drugs and Chemicals, Acetaminophen, Poisoning, Accidental (unintentional). Review the Tabular for the correct seventh character.
R11.2 Nausea (without vomiting), with vomiting

**1.143.** R11.2 Nausea, with vomiting
R53.83 Fatigue
T46.0X5A Table of Drugs and Chemicals, Digoxin, adverse effect

**1.144.** I13.2     Disease, diseased, heart (organic), hypertensive – *see* Hypertension, heart. Hypertension, hypertensive (accelerated) (benign) (essential) (idiopathic) (malignant) (systemic), heart (disease) with kidney disease (chronic) – *see* Hypertension, cardiorenal (disease), with heart failure, with stage 5 or end stage renal disease

        I50.9     Failure, heart (acute) (sudden), congestive (compensated) (decompensated). The "use additional code" statement under code I13.2 indicates the use of this code to identify the type of heart failure.

        N18.5     Disease, diseased, kidney (functional) (pelvis), chronic, stage 5. (The "use additional code" statement under code I13.2 indicates the use of this code to identify the stage of the chronic kidney disease.)

        T50.1X6A     Refer to Table of Drugs and Chemicals, Lasix, underdosing

        Z91.130     Noncompliance, with, medication regimen, underdosing, unintentional, due to patient's age-related debility

**1.145.** I49.5     Syndrome, sick, sinus

        T82.110A     Complication(s) (from) (of), cardiovascular device, graft, or implant, electronic, electrode, mechanical, breakdown. Review the Tabular for assignment of seventh character.

        Z53.8     Canceled procedure (surgical), because of, specified reason NEC

**1.146.** T84.51XA     Complication(s) (from) (of), joint prosthesis, internal, infection or inflammation, hip. Review the Tabular for complete code assignment and seventh character.

**1.147.** S22.41XA     Fracture, traumatic (abduction) (adduction) (separation), rib, multiple. Review the Tabular for complete code assignment and correct seventh character.

        S62.101A     Fracture, traumatic (abduction) (adduction) (separation), wrist. Review the Tabular for complete code assignment and correct seventh character.

**1.148.** T40.7X2A     Table of Drugs and Chemicals, Marijuana, Poisoning, Intentional, Self-harm. Review the Tabular for seventh character.

        T40.5X2A     Table of Drugs and Chemicals, Cocaine, Poisoning, Intentional, Self-harm. Review the Tabular for seventh character.

        S01.412A     Laceration, cheek (external). Review the Tabular for complete code assignment and seventh character.

        S01.01XA     Laceration, scalp. Review the Tabular for complete code assignment and seventh character.

## *Chapter 20 Coding Cases*

**1.149.** V43.53XA     Index to External Causes, Accident, car – *see* Accident, transport, car occupant. Accident, transport, car occupant, driver, collision (with) pickup truck (traffic)

        Y92.411     Index to External Causes, Place of occurrence, highway (interstate)

        Y93.C2     Index to External Causes, Activity (involving) (of victim at time of event), cellular, telephone

**1.150.** Y37.230A    Index to External Causes, Military operations (injuries to military and civilians occurring during peacetime on military property and during routine military exercises and operations) (by) (from) (involving) explosion (of) improvised explosive device [IED] (person-borne) (roadside) (vehicle-borne)

Y92.139    Index to External Causes, Place of occurrence, military base – *see* Place of occurrence, residence, institutional, military base

Y99.1    Index to External Causes, External cause status, military activity

**1.151.** W54.0XXA    Index to External Causes, Bite, bitten by, dog

Y92.71    Index to External Causes, Place of occurrence, barn

Y93.K9    Index to External Causes, Activity (involving) (of victim at time of event), animal care NEC

Y99.0    Index to External Causes, External cause status, civilian activity done for income or pay

**1.152.** X10.2XXA    Index to External Causes, Burn, burned, burning (accidental) (by) (from) (on), hot, oil (cooking)

Y92.511    Index to External Causes, Place of occurrence, restaurant

Y93.G3    Index to External Causes, Activity (involving) (of victim at time of event), cooking and baking

Y99.0    Index to External Causes, External cause status, civilian activity done for income or pay

**1.153.** S72.002A    Fracture, traumatic (abduction) (adduction) (separation) femur, femoral, neck – *see* fracture, femur, upper end, neck

W11.XXXA    Index to External Causes, Fall, falling (accidental), from, off, out of, ladder

Y92.018    Index to External Causes, Place of occurrence, residence (non-institutional) (private), house, single family, specified NEC

Y93.H9    Index to External Causes, Activity (involving) (of victim at time of event), maintenance, property

Y99.8    Index to External Causes, External cause status, specified NEC

**1.154.** S32.019D    Fracture, traumatic (abduction) (adduction) (separation) vertebra, vertebral (arch) (body) (column) (neural arch) (pedicle) (spinous process) (transverse process), lumbar, first

S32.029D    Fracture, vertebra, vertebral (arch) (body) (column) (neural arch) (pedicle) (spinous process) (transverse process), lumbar, second

W11.XXXD    Index to External Causes, Fall, falling (accidental), from ladder

**1.155.** T24.332A    Burn (electricity) (flame) (hot gas, liquid or hot object) (radiation) (steam) (thermal), calf, left, third degree

T21.34XA    Burn (electricity) (flame) (hot gas, liquid or hot object) (radiation) (steam) (thermal), back, third degree

X02.0XXA    Index to External Causes, Fall, falling (accidental), into, fire – *see* Exposure, fire, by type. Exposure (to), fire, flames (accidental) fireplace, furnace or stove – *see* Exposure, fire, controlled, building. Exposure, fire, flames (accidental), controlled (in), building or structure

Y92.003    Index to External Causes, Place of occurrence, residence (non-institutional) (private), bedroom

Y93.02    Index to External Causes, Activity (involving) (of victim at time of event), running

Y99.8    Index to External Causes, External cause status, specified NEC

**1.156.** T22.212D    Burn, (electricity) (flame) (hot gas, liquid or hot object) (radiation) (steam) (thermal) forearm, left, second degree

X10.2XXD    Index to External Causes, Burn, burned, burning (accidental) (by) (from) (on), hot, fat

Z48.00    Change(s) (in) (of) dressing (nonsurgical)

**1.157.** S52.301B    Fracture, traumatic (abduction) (adduction) (separation), radius, shaft. Review tabular for complete code assignment

S52.201B    Fracture, traumatic (abduction) (adduction) (separation), ulna, shaft. Review the Tabular for complete code assignment.

S16.1XXA    Strain, cervical

V43.52XA    Index to External Causes, Accident (to), car – *see* Accident, transport, car occupant, driver, collision (with), car (traffic)

Y92.411    Index to External Causes, Place of occurrence, street and highway, interstate highway

**1.158.** S42.401K    Nonunion, fracture – *see* fracture, by site. Fracture, traumatic, humerus, distal end – *see* Fracture, humerus, lower end, lower end

V00.121D    Index to External Causes, Fall, falling (accidental), involving, skates (ice) (in line) (roller) – *see* Accident, transport, pedestrian, conveyance, roller skates (non in-line), fall

**1.159.** L08.9    Infection, infected, infective, skin (Local) (staphylococcal) (streptococcal)

S61.411A    Wound, open, hand, laceration – *see* laceration, hand, right

W25.XXXA    Index to External Causes, Cut, cutting (any part of body) (accidental) – *see also* Contact, with, glass (sharp) (broken)

Y92.511    Index to External Causes, Place of occurrence, restaurant

F10.10    Abuse, alcohol

F15.10    Abuse, amphetamine (or related substance) – *see* Abuse, drug, stimulant NEC

Y99.8    Index to External Causes, External cause status, leisure activity

**1.160.** S06.9X2A    Injury, head, with loss of consciousness. Review Tabular for complete code assignment.

R40.2121    Coma, with, opening of eyes, in response to, pain

R40.2211    Coma, with verbal response (none)

R40.2311    Coma, with motor response (none)

Y04.0XXA    Index to External Causes, Assault (homicidal) (by) (in), fight (hand) (fists) (foot) (unarmed)

Y92.830    Index to External Causes, Place of occurrence, recreation area, park (public)

Y93.01    Index to External Causes, Activity (involving) (of victim at time of event), walking (on level or elevated terrain)

Y99.8    Index to External Causes, External cause status, student activity

**1.161.** S02.10XA    Fracture, traumatic (abduction) (adduction) (separation), skull, base

S06.5X0A    Hematoma (traumatic) (skin surface intact), subdural (traumatic) – *see* Injury, intracranial (traumatic), subdural hemorrhage, traumatic. Review Tabular for complete code assignment.

S82.855A    Fracture, traumatic, trimalleolar – *see* fracture, ankle, trimalleolar, nondisplaced. Review Tabular for complete code assignment.

W00.1XXA    Index to External Causes, Fall, falling (accidental) due to, ice or snow, from one level to another, on stairs or steps

Y92.018    Index to External Causes, Place of occurrence, residence (non-institutional) (private) house, single family, specified NEC

Y99.8    Index to External Causes, External cause status, specified NEC

**1.162.** S12.100A     Fracture, traumatic, vertebra, vertebral (arch) (body) (column) (neural arch) (pedicle) (spinous process) (transverse process), cervical, second (axis) – *see* Fracture, neck, cervical vertebra, second (displaced)

      S14.112A     Injury, spinal (cord), cervical (neck), complete lesion, C2 level

      S06.9X1A     Injury, head, with loss of consciousness. Review Tabular for complete code assignment.

      V20.4XXA     Index to External Causes, Accident, transport, motorcyclist, driver, collision (with), animal (traffic)

      Y92.410     Index to External Causes, Place of occurrence, street and highway

      Y99.8     Index to External Causes, External cause status, leisure activity

## *Chapter 21 Coding Cases*

**1.163.** Z38.00     Newborn (infant) (liveborn) (singleton) born in hospital

      P55.0     Incompatibility, Rh (blood group) (factor), newborn

      Z67.10     Blood, type, A (Rh positive)

**1.164.** Z02.0     Examination (for) (following) (general) (of) (routine), medical (adult) (for) (of) preschool children, for admission to school

**1.165.** Z44.121     Encounter (with health service) (for) fitting (of) – *see* Fitting (and adjustment) (of). Fitting (and adjustment) (of) artificial, leg – *see* Admission, adjustment, artificial, leg. Admission (for), adjustment (of), artificial, leg, partial

      Z89.511     Absence (of) (organ or part) (complete or partial) leg (acquired) (above knee), below knee (acquired)

**1.166.** M81.0     Osteoporosis (female) (male), postmenopausal

      Z87.310     History, personal (of), fracture (healed) osteoporosis

**1.167.** I21.29     Infarct, infarction, myocardium, myocardial (acute) (with stated duration of 4 weeks or less), ST elevation (STEMI), lateral (apical-lateral) (basal-lateral) (high)

      Z92.82     Status (post), administration of tPA (rtPA) in a different facility within the last 24 hours prior to admission to current facility

**1.168.** Z43.6     Attention (to), artificial opening (of), urinary tract NEC

      Z90.6     Absence (of) (organ or part) (complete or partial), bladder (acquired)

      Z85.51     History, personal (of), malignant neoplasm (of), bladder

**1.169.** S32.411D     Fracture, traumatic (abduction) (adduction) (separation), acetabulum, wall, anterior

      V03.90XD     Index to External Causes, Accident (to), pedestrian (on foot), with, transport vehicle – *see* Accident, transport, pedestrian, on foot, collision (with), car

# Part II: Site-Specific Cases

## Long-Term Care Cases

**1.170.** N39.0     Infection, infected, infective (opportunistic) urinary (tract)

B96.20     Infection, infected, infective (opportunistic) bacterial, as cause of disease classified elsewhere, Escherichia coli [E. coli]

Z79.2     Long-term, (current) (prophylactic), drug therapy (use of), antibiotics

G35     Sclerosis, sclerotic, multiple (brain stem) (cerebral) (generalized) (spinal cord)

**1.171.** S52.92XE     Fracture, traumatic (abduction) (adduction) (separation), radius

S52.202E     Fracture, traumatic (abduction) (adduction) (separation), ulna (shaft)

X58.XXXD     Index to External Causes, Accident (to)

**1.172.** Z48.812     Aftercare, following surgery (for) (on), circulatory system

Z95.1     Status (post), aortocoronary bypass

G89.12     Pain(s) (see also Painful), acute, post-thoracotomy

**1.173.** G35     Sclerosis, sclerotic, multiple (brain stem) (cerebral) (generalized) (spinal cord)

S32.9XXD     Fracture, traumatic, (abduction) (adduction) (separation), pelvis, pelvic (bone)

V00.811D     Index to External Causes, Fall, falling (accidental) from, wheelchair, powered – see Accident, transport, pedestrian, conveyance occupant, specified type NEC, wheelchair (powered), fall

**1.174.** Z45.02     Admission (for), adjustment, device NEC, implanted, cardiac, defibrillator, or Encounter, (with health service) (for) adjustment and management (of), implanted device

I49.01     Fibrillation, ventricular

I25.10     Disease, diseased, coronary (artery) – see Disease, heart (organic), ischemic, atherosclerotic (of)

**1.175.** S63.004A     Dislocation (articular), wrist (carpal bone)

W18.30XA     Index to External Causes, Fall, falling (accidental) same level

Y92.128     Index to External Causes, Place of occurrence, residence, institutional, nursing home, specified NEC

Y93.01     Index to External Causes, Activity (involving) (of victim at time of event), walking (on level or elevated terrain)

Y99.8     Index to External Causes, External cause status, leisure activity

**1.176.** G20     Disease, Parkinson's

E10.9     Diabetes, type 1

J44.9     Disease, pulmonary, chronic obstructive

Z60.2     Living alone (problems with)

**1.177.** R19.7     Diarrhea, diarrheal (disease) (infantile) (inflammatory)

R11.0     Nausea (without vomiting)

T45.1X5D     Table of Drugs and Chemicals, Fluorouracil, adverse effect column

C18.4     Carcinoma – see also Neoplasm, by site, malignant
Neoplasm Table, intestine, large, colon, transverse, in Malignant Primary column

**1.178.** Z48.01    Aftercare, following surgery, attention to dressings, surgical
         Z89.512   Absence (of) (organ or part) (complete or partial), extremity (acquired), lower, below knee

**1.179.** R40.20    Coma
         T42.4X2S  Late effect(s) – *see* Sequelae, poisoning – code to poisoning with seventh character S. Table of Drugs and Chemicals, valium, poisoning-intentional self-harm
         T51.0X2S  Late effect(s) – *see* Sequelae, poisoning – code to poisoning with seventh character S. Table of Drugs and Chemicals, alcohol, beverage, poisoning-intentional self-harm

**1.180.** M80.021D  Osteoporosis (female) (male), senile – *see* Osteoporosis, age-related, with current pathologic fracture, humerus

**1.181.** K51.90    Colitis (acute) (catarrhal) (chronic) (noninfective) (hemorrhagic), ulcerative (chronic)
         M81.8     Osteoporosis (female) (male), drug-induced – *see* Osteoporosis, specified type NEC
         T38.0X5S  Table of Drugs and Chemicals, corticosteroids, adverse effect
         Z79.52    Long-term (current) (prophylactic) drug therapy (use of), steroids, systemic

**1.182.** M86.171   Osteomyelitis (general) (infective) (localized) (neonatal) (purulent) (septic) (staphylococcal) (streptococcal) (suppurative) (with periostitis), acute, tarsus
         I96       Gangrene, gangrenous (connective tissue) (dropsical) (dry) (moist) (skin) (ulcer), extremity (lower) (upper)
         L89.513   Ulcer, ulcerated, ulcerating, ulceration, ulcerative, decubitus – *see* Ulcer, pressure, by site, pressure (pressure area), ankle
         E10.51    Diabetes, diabetic (mellitus) (sugar), type 1, with, peripheral angiopathy
         I12.9     Disease, diseased, kidney (functional) (pelvis), chronic, hypertensive – *see* Hypertension, kidney. Hypertension, hypertensive (accelerated) (benign) (essential) (idiopathic) (malignant) (systemic), kidney, with, stage 1 through stage 4 chronic kidney disease
         N18.4     Disease, diseased, kidney (functional) (pelvis), chronic, stage 4 (severe)
         Z89.512   Absence (of) (organ or part) (complete or partial), limb (acquired) – *see* Absence, extremity (acquired), lower, below knee
         E78.0     Hypercholesterolemia (essential) (familial) (hereditary) (primary) (pure)
         F10.21    Alcoholism (chronic), with remission

**1.183.** I50.9     Failure, failed, heart (acute) (senile) (sudden) congestive (compensated) (decompensated)
         I48.91    Fibrillation, atrial or auricular (established)
         S72.012D  Fracture, traumatic (abduction) (adduction) (separation), femur, femoral, neck, *see* Fracture, femur, upper end, subcapital (displaced)
         W06.XXXD  Index to External Causes, Fall, falling (accidental) from, off, out of, bed

**1.184.** I69.354   Hemiplegia, following, cerebrovascular disease, cerebral infarction, <u>or</u> Sequelae (of), infarction, cerebral, hemiplegia
         I69.321   Dysphasia, following, cerebrovascular disease, cerebral infarction <u>or</u> Sequelae (of), infarction, cerebral, dysphasia
         I69.392   Sequelae (of), infarction, cerebral, facial droop
         K21.9     Disease, diseased, gastroesophageal reflux (GERD)
         M06.9     Arthritis, arthritic (acute) (chronic) (nonpyogenic) (subacute), rheumatoid
         G30.0     Disease, diseased, Alzheimer's, early onset, with behavioral disturbance
         F02.81

**1.185.** I69.352    Hemiplegia, following, cerebrovascular disease, cerebral infarction, <u>or</u> Sequelae (of), infarction, cerebral, hemiplegia

I69.398    Alteration (of), altered, sensation, following, cerebrovascular disease, cerebral infarction, <u>or</u> Sequelae, infarction, cerebral, specified effect

R43.9    Sense loss, taste – *see* Disturbance(s), sensation, taste

**1.186.** G30.0    Disease, diseased, Alzheimer's, early onset, with behavioral disturbance
F02.81

I63.40    Infarct, infarction, cerebral, due to embolism, cerebral arteries

G81.91    Hemiplegia. Review Tabular for complete code assignment.

R47.01    Aphasia (amnestic) (global) (nominal) (semantic) (syntactic)

Z91.83    Wandering, in diseases classified elsewhere

**1.187.** J15.1    Pneumonia, in (due to) Pseudomonas

G20    Dementia (degenerative) (primary) (old age) (persisting), in (due to) Parkinson's disease (Parkinsonism)

F02.80

I34.0    Regurgitation, mitral (valve) – *see* Insufficiency, mitral. Insufficiency, insufficient, mitral (valve)

M40.209    Kyphosis, kyphotic (acquired)

J45.909    Asthma, asthmatic (bronchial) (catarrh) (spasmodic)

E11.9    Diabetes, diabetic (mellitus) (sugar) type 2

**1.188.** T84.50XD    Complication(s) (from) (of), joint prosthesis, internal, infection or inflammation, hip. Review Tabular for complete code assignment.

B95.2    Infection, infected, infective (opportunistic), bacterial, as cause of disease classified elsewhere, enterococcus

Z16.21    Resistance, resistant, organism (s), to, drug, vancomycin

Z95.828    Presence (of), vascular implant or device, access port device
Hypertrophy, prostate – *see* Enlargement, enlarged, prostate

N40.1    Enlargement, enlarged, prostate, with lower urinary tract symptoms (LUTS

N13.8    Obstruction, obstructed, obstructive, urinary, specified NEC

F43.24    Depression (acute) (mental), situational

I10    Hypertension, hypertensive (accelerated) (benign) (essential) (idiopathic) (malignant) (systemic)

I48.91    Fibrillation, atrial or auricular (established)

Z79.01    Long-term (current) (prophylactic) drug therapy (use of) anticoagulants

Z51.81    Monitoring (encounter for), therapeutic drug level

**1.189.** Z47.81    Aftercare, following surgery (for) (on), amputation

E11.51    Diabetes, diabetic (mellitus) (sugar), type 2, with peripheral angiopathy

E11.43    Diabetes, diabetic (mellitus) (sugar), type 2, with gastroparesis

I08.0    Regurgitation, mitral (valve) – *see* Insufficiency, mitral. Insufficiency, insufficient, mitral (valve), with aortic valve disease

K40.90    Hernia, hernial (acquired) (recurrent), inguinal (direct) (external) (funicular) (indirect) (internal) (oblique) (scrotal) (sliding)

M15.9    Disease, diseased, joint, degenerative – *see* Osteoarthritis. Osteoarthritis, generalized

J44.9    Disease, diseased, pulmonary, chronic obstructive

Z79.4    Long-term (current) (prophylactic) drug therapy (use of) insulin

Z89.439    Absence (of ) (organ or part) (complete or partial), foot (acquired)

## *Home Healthcare Cases*

**1.190.** S01.81XD    Laceration, face – *see* Laceration, head, specified site
      X58.XXXD    Index to External Causes, Accident (to)

**1.191.** Z48.812    Aftercare, following surgery (for) (on), circulatory system
      Z48.01    Aftercare, following surgery (for) (on), attention to, dressings, surgical
      I25.10    Atherosclerosis, coronary artery
      Z95.0    Status (post), pacemaker, cardiac

**1.192.** T78.40XA    Allergy, allergic (reaction) (to). Review Tabular for complete code assignment.
      T45.1X5A    Allergy, allergic (reaction) (to), drug, medicament & biological (any) (external) (internal), correct substance properly administered – *see* Table of Drugs and Chemicals, by drug, adverse effect, fluorouracil
      C80.1    Cancer, unspecified site (primary) (secondary)

**1.193.** S72.21XD    Aftercare, fracture – code to fracture with seventh character D. Fracture, traumatic, hip – *see* Fracture, femur, neck. Fracture, femur, neck – *see* Fracture, femur, upper end, neck. Fracture, femur, upper end, subtrochanteric (displaced)
      Z48.01    Admission (for), change of, surgical dressing
      W10.0XXD    Index to External Causes, Fall, falling, from, off, out of, escalator

**1.194.** Z47.1    Aftercare, following surgery (for) (on), joint replacement
      Z96.642    Status (post), organ replacement, by artificial or mechanical device or prosthesis of, joint, hip – *see* Presence, hip joint implant. Presence (of), hip-joint implant (artificial) (functional) (prosthesis)
      R26.2    Gait, abnormality, walking difficulty NEC
      Z51.81    Monitoring (encounter for), therapeutic drug level
      Z79.01    Therapy, drug, long-term (current) (prophylactic), anticoagulants
      Z48.01    Change(s) (in) (of), dressing, surgical

**1.195.** J44.9    Disease, diseased, pulmonary, chronic obstructive
      Z99.81    Dependence (on) (syndrome), oxygen (long term) (supplemental)

**1.196.** L03.113    Cellulitis (diffuse) (phlegmonous) (septic) (suppurative), upper limb. Review Tabular for complete code assignment
      Z79.2    Long-term (current) (prophylactic) drug therapy (use of), antibiotics
      Z45.2    Admission (for), adjustment (of), device, vascular access

**1.197.** Z48.3    Aftercare, following surgery (for) (on), neoplasm
      C50.511    Refer to Neoplasm Table, by site (breast), malignant, primary site, lower-outer quadrant. Review Tabular for complete code assignment.
      Z48.01    Admission (for), change of, surgical dressing
      Z90.11    Absence (of) (organ or part) (complete or partial), breast(s) (and nipple(s)) (acquired)

**1.198.** Z47.1    Aftercare, following surgery (for) (on), joint replacement
      Z96.651    Status (post), organ replacement, by artificial or mechanical device or prosthesis of, joint, knee – *see* Presence (of), knee joint implant (functional) (prosthesis)
      R26.9    Abnormality, gait – *see* Gait. Gait abnormality

**1.199.** Z47.1      Aftercare, following surgery (for) (on), joint replacement

       T81.4XXA      Infection, infected, infective (opportunistic), postoperative wound. Review Tabular for complete code assignment.

       R26.9      Abnormality, gait – *see* Gait. Gait abnormality

       Z48.01      Aftercare, following surgery, attention to dressings, surgical

       Z96.642      Status (post), organ replacement, by artificial or mechanical device or prosthesis of, joint, hip – *see* Presence (of), hip joint implant (functional) (prosthesis)

**1.200.** Z46.6      Admission (for), adjustment (of), device, urinary <u>or</u> Change(s) (in) (of), indwelling catheter

       N31.9      Neurogenic, bladder

**1.201.** Z48.815      Aftercare, following surgery (for) (on), digestive system

       Z48.01      Aftercare, following surgery (for) (on), attention to dressings, surgical

       Z48.03      Aftercare, following surgery (for) (on), attention to drains

**1.202.** I50.9      Failure, failed, heart (acute) (senile) (sudden), congestive (compensated) (decompensated)

       I73.9      Insufficiency, insufficient, vascular, peripheral

       E03.9      Hypothyroidism (acquired)

**1.203.** E10.65      Diabetes, diabetic (mellitus) (sugar), poorly controlled – code to Diabetes, by type, with hyperglycemia, type 1

       Z71.3      Counseling (for), dietary

       Z46.81      Counseling (for), insulin pump use, <u>or</u>

             Encounter (with health service) (for), training, insulin pump

**1.204.** Z48.812      Aftercare, following surgery (for) (on), circulatory system

       I25.10      Disease, diseased, coronary (artery) – *see* Disease, heart (organic), ischemic, atherosclerotic (of)

       Z95.1      Status (post), aortocoronary bypass

**1.205.** Z48.3      Aftercare, following surgery (for) (on), neoplasm

       C18.7      Neoplasm Table, by site, intestine, large, colon, sigmoid (flexure) in Malignant Primary column

       Z43.3      Colostomy, attention to

**1.206.** S72.002D      Fracture, traumatic (abduction) (adduction) (separation), hip – *see* Fracture, traumatic, femur, upper end, neck

       R26.9      Abnormality, gait – *see* Gait. Gait abnormality

       W19.XXXD      Fall, falling (accidental)

**1.207.** T81.4XXD      Infection, infected, infective, postoperative wound

       Z47.1      Aftercare, following surgery (for) (on), joint replacement

       T81.31XD      Dehiscence (of), operation wound, external operation wound (superficial)

       B95.62      Infection, infected, infective, staphylococcal, as cause of disease classified elsewhere, aureus, methicillin resistant (MRSA) <u>or</u> MRSA, infection, as the cause of diseases classified elsewhere

       Z96.642      Presence (of), implanted device, joint, hip

       M15.9      Osteoarthritis, generalized

       R26.9      Abnormality, gait – *see* Gait. Gait abnormality

**1.208.** Z48.3      Aftercare, following surgery (for) (on), neoplasm
       C50.911      Neoplasm Table, by site (breast), malignant primary column
       I69.398      Sequelae (of), stroke, specified effect NEC
       M62.81      Weak, weakening, weakness (generalized), muscle
       Z90.11      Absence (of) (organ or part) (complete or partial), breast(s) (nipple(s)) (acquired)

**1.209.** I69.341      Monoplegia, following, cerebrovascular disease, cerebral infarction, lower limb <u>or</u> Sequelae, infarction, cerebral, monoplegia, lower limb
       R26.9      Abnormality, gait – *see* Gait. Gait abnormality
       Z99.3      Status (post), wheelchair confinement

## *Hospital Inpatient Cases*

**1.210.** A41.51      Sepsis (generalized), Escherichia coli (E. coli)
       N39.0      Infection, infected, infective (opportunistic), urinary (tract)
       B95.1      Infection, infected, infective (opportunistic), bacterial NOS, as cause of disease classified elsewhere, streptococcus, group B
       B96.20      Infection, infected, infective (opportunistic), bacterial NOS, as cause of disease classified elsewhere, Escherichia coli [E. coli]
       J44.9      Disease, diseased, pulmonary, chronic obstructive
       I69.920      Aphasia (amnestic) (global) (nominal) (semantic) (syntactic) following, cerebrovascular disease
       I69.951      Sequelae (of), disease, cerebrovascular, hemiplegia
       N28.9      Insufficiency, insufficient, renal (acute)

**1.211.** D64.81      Anemia (essential) (general) (hemoglobin deficiency) (infantile) (primary) (profound), due to (in) (with), antineoplastic chemotherapy
       C25.0      Carcinoma (malignant) – *see also* Neoplasm Table, by site, malignant Neoplasm Table, Pancreas, head, malignant primary column
       T45.1X5A      Table of Drugs and Chemicals, Antineoplastic NEC

**1.212.** C79.31      Neoplasm Table, by site, (brain NEC), secondary
       C80.1      Neoplasm Table, by site (unknown site or unspecified), malignant primary
       G30.1      Disease, diseased, Alzheimer's, late onset
       F02.80
       S00.83XA      Contusion (skin surface intact), head, specified part NEC
       F32.9      Depression (acute) (mental)
       J43.9      Emphysema (atrophic) (bullous) (chronic) (interlobular) (lung) (obstructive) (pulmonary) (senile) (vesicular)
       W05.0XXA      Index to External Causes, Fall, falling (accidental) from, off, out of, wheelchair, non-moving
       Y92.129      Index to External Causes, Place of Occurrence, residence, institutional, nursing home
       Y99.8      Index to External Causes, External cause status, specified NEC

**1.213.** E11.649      Diabetes, diabetic (mellitus) (sugar), type 2, with hypoglycemia
       C34.11      Neoplasm Table, by site, (lung), upper lobe malignant, primary
       E11.21      Diabetes, diabetic (mellitus) (sugar), type 2, with nephropathy
       E11.40      Diabetes, diabetic (mellitus) (sugar), type 2, with neuropathy

       R16.0      Hepatomegaly, *see also* Hypertrophy, liver
                      Hypertrophy, hypertrophic, liver
       E78.5      Hyperlipemia, hyperlipidemia
       Z79.4      Long-term (current) (prophylactic), drug therapy (use of), insulin

**1.214.** I50.9      Failure, failed, heart (acute) (senile) (sudden), congestive (compensated) (decompensated)

       E86.0      Dehydration

       D69.49      Thrombocytopenia, thrombocytopenic, primary NEC

       N39.0      Infection, infected, infective (opportunistic), urinary (tract)

       E11.9      Diabetes, diabetic (mellitus) (sugar), type 2

**1.215.** I11.0      Hypertension, hypertensive, heart, with, heart failure (congestive)

       I50.1      Failure, failed, heart (acute) (senile) (sudden), with, acute pulmonary edema – *see* Failure, ventricular, left

       J15.1      Pneumonia, in (due to) Pseudomonas NEC

       J44.9      Disease, diseased, pulmonary, chronic obstructive

       Z87.891      History, personal (of), nicotine dependence

       Z66      Status (post), do not resuscitate (DNR)

**1.216.** J18.1      Pneumonia, lobar (disseminated) (double) (interstitial)

       I50.33      Failure, failed, heart (acute) (senile) (sudden), diastolic (congestive), acute (congestive), and (on) chronic (congestive)

       I10      Hypertension, hypertensive

       I20.9      Angina

       F41.9      Anxiety

       I25.2      Infarct, Infarction, myocardium, myocardial, healed or old

**1.217.** O24.410      Pregnancy (single) (uterine), complicated by (care of) (management affected by), diabetes (mellitus), gestational (pregnancy induced) – *see* Diabetes, gestational
Diabetes, diabetic (mellitus) (sugar), gestational (in pregnancy), diet controlled

       O99.89      Pregnancy (single) (uterine), complicated by (care of) (management affected by), disorders of, specified NEC

       M62.08      Diastasis, muscle, specified site NEC

       Z3A.40      Pregnancy (single) (uterine), weeks of gestation, 40 weeks

**1.218.** P38.9      Omphalitis (congenital) (newborn)

       B95.62      Infection, infected, infective (opportunistic), staphylococcal NEC, as cause of disease classified elsewhere, aureus, methicillin resistant (MRSA)

       B95.4      Infection, infected, infective (opportunistic), bacterial NOS, as cause of disease classified elsewhere, Streptococcus, specified NEC

**1.219.** T43.622A      Overdose, overdosage (drug) – *see* Table of Drugs and Chemicals, by drug, poisoning. Table of Drugs and Chemicals, Amphetamines, NEC

       T51.0X2A      Overdose, overdosage (drug), – *see* Table of Drugs and Chemicals, by drug, poisoning. Table of Drugs and Chemicals, Alcohol, beverage

       F10.229      Dependence (on) (syndrome) alcohol (ethyl) (methyl) (without remission), with, intoxication

       F15.229      Dependence (on) (syndrome), amphetamine(s) (type) *see* Dependence, drug, stimulant, NEC, with, intoxication

       R00.0      Tachycardia

       F90.9      Disorder (of), attention-deficit hyperactivity (adolescent) (adult) (child)

       F91.1      Disorder (of), aggressive, unsocialized

       E86.0      Dehydration

       Y90.2      Index to External Causes, Blood alcohol level, 40–59 mg/100 ml

**1.220.** T84.032A    Complication(s) (from) (of), joint prosthesis, internal, mechanical, loosening, knee. Review the Tabular for complete code assignment.

G20    Parkinsonism (idiopathic) (primary)

I11.0    Hypertension, hypertensive, heart (disease), with heart failure (congestive)

I50.9    Failure, failed, heart, congestive

H40.1430    Glaucoma, capsular – *see* Glaucoma, open angle, primary, capsular. See Tabular for complete code assignment.

I25.2    Infarct, Infarction, myocardium, myocardial, healed or old

R94.39    Findings, abnormal, inconclusive, without diagnosis, stress test

**1.221.** D25.0    Leiomyoma, uterus (cervix) (corpus), submucous

N80.0    Endometriosis, uterus (internal)

N80.1    Endometriosis, ovary

N80.3    Endometriosis, pelvic peritoneum

N73.6    Adhesions, adhesive, peritoneum, peritoneal, pelvic, female

K91.72    Complication(s) (from) (of), intraoperative (intraprocedural), puncture or laceration (accidental) (unintentional) (of), digestive system, during procedure on other organ

D62    Anemia, blood loss, acute

Y92.234    Index to External Causes, Place of occurrence, hospital, operating room

**1.222.** Z38.00    Newborn

Q25.1    Coarctation of aorta (preductal) (postductal)

Q21.0    Defect, defective, ventricular septal

Q69.1    Polydactylism

Q66.89    Deformity, foot, congenital, specified type NEC

Q68.1    Deformity, hand, congenital

## *Physician-Related Cases*

**1.223.** D27.1    Sertoli-Leydig cell tumor – *see* Neoplasm, benign. Neoplasm, neoplastic – *see* also Neoplasm Table. Neoplasm Table, ovary, benign column. Review the Tabular for complete code assignment.

**1.224.** R76.11    Findings, abnormal, inconclusive, without diagnosis, tuberculin skin test (without active tuberculosis)

G70.00    Myasthenia gravis

M41.124    Scoliosis (acquired) (postural), adolescent (idiopathic) *see* Scoliosis, idiopathic, thoracic

**1.225.** Z01.419    Examination (for) (following) (general) (of) (routine), annual (adult) (periodic) (physical), gynecological

M1A.9XX1    Gout, chronic

Z23    Vaccination (prophylactic), encounter for

**1.226.** C71.7    Ependymoma (epithelial) (malignant), specified site – *see* Neoplasm, malignant. Neoplasm Table, Brain, midbrain, primary

G97.48    Complications (from) (of), intraoperative (intraprocedural), puncture or laceration (accidental) (unintentional) (of), brain, during a nervous system procedure

M62.81    Weak, weakening, weakness (generalized), muscle

Y92.234    Index to External Causes, Place of occurrence, hospital, operating room

**1.227.** A69.23      Arthritis, arthritic, (acute) (chronic) (nonpyogenic) (subacute) due to or associated with Lyme disease

       S40.861S      Bite(s), (animal) (human), arm (upper), superficial NEC, insect. Review the Tabular for complete code assignment.

       E66.01      Obesity, morbid

       Z68.41      Body, bodies, mass index (BMI), adult, 40–44.9

       W57.XXXS      Index to External Causes, Bite, bitten by, insect, (nonvenomous)

**1.228.** D21.22      Fibroma - *see also* Neoplasm, connective tissue, benign. Neoplasm Table, Connective tissue, foot, benign

       D21.21      Neoplasm Table, Connective tissue, foot, benign column

       E11.40      Diabetes, diabetic, (mellitus) (sugar), type 2 with neuropathy

**1.229.** Z30.2      Multiparity (grand), requiring contraceptive management – *see* Contraception. Contraception, contraceptive, sterilization

       N90.89      Tag (hypertrophied skin) (infected), vulva

**1.230.** K12.2      Cellulitis (diffuse) (phlegmonous) (septic) (suppurative), mouth (floor)

       K12.0      Ulcer, ulcerated, ulcerating, ulceration, ulcerative, aphthous (oral) (recurrent)

       B08.5      Herpangina

**1.231.** B37.3      Candidiasis, candidal, vagina

       B35.4      Tinea (intersecta) (tarsi) corporis

       E28.2      Syndrome, ovary, polycystic

**1.232.** S83.231A      Tear, torn (traumatic) meniscus (knee) (current injury), medial, complex

       M71.21      Baker's cyst – *see* Cyst, Baker's

       M22.41      Chondromalacia (systemic), patella

       W19.XXXA      Index to External Causes, Fall, falling (accidental)

       Y92.830      Index to External Causes, Place of occurrence, park (public)

       Y93.02      Index to External Causes, Activity (involving) running

       Y99.8      Index to External Causes, External cause status, leisure activity

**1.233.** C78.7      Carcinoma – *see also* Neoplasm by site, malignant. Neoplasm Table – liver, malignant secondary column

       Z85.068      History, personal (of), malignant neoplasm (of), small intestine

       Z66      Status (post), do not resuscitate (DNR)

       Z90.49      Absence (of) (organ or part) (complete or partial), duodenum (acquired)

       Z92.21      History, personal (of), chemotherapy for neoplastic condition

**1.234.** F90.2      Disorder (of), attention-deficit hyperactivity (adolescent) (adult) (child), combined type

       F82      Disorder (of), developmental, coordination (motor)

**1.235.** Q77.4      Achondroplasia (osteosclerosis congenita) <u>or</u> Osteosclerosis congenita

       G47.33      Apnea, apneic (spells) sleep, obstructive (adult) (pediatric)

       Q76.426      Lordosis, congenital, lumbar region

       Z82.79      History, family (of), chromosomal anomaly <u>or</u>
History, family (of), congenital malformations and deformations

**1.236.** H81.02      Vertigo, labyrinthine – *see* subcategory H81.0

       R51      Headache

**1.237.** R51      Pain(s) (*see also* Painful), face, facial
R68.84     Pain(s) (*see also* Painful), jaw
G51.0      Bell's palsy, paralysis, <u>or</u> Palsy, Bell's – *see also* Palsy, facial
H65.92     Otitis (acute), media (hemorrhagic) (staphylococcal) (streptococcal), nonsuppurative

**1.238.** L03.012   Paronychia – *see also* Cellulitis, digit
Cellulitis (diffuse) (phlegmonous) (septic) (suppurative), digit, finger – *see* Cellulitis, finger (intrathecal) (periosteal) (subcutaneous) (subcuticular)
J41.0      Cough (affected) (chronic) (epidemic) (nervous), smokers'
Z72.0      Tobacco (nicotine), use

**1.239.** O99.283  Pregnancy (single) (uterine), complicated by (care of) (management affected by), endocrine diseases
O24.410  Diabetes, diabetic (mellitus) (sugar), gestational (in pregnancy), diet controlled
E06.3      Thyroiditis, Hashimoto's (struma lymphomatosa)
Z3A.34    Pregnancy (single) (uterine), weeks of gestation, 34 weeks

**1.240.** M79.641  Pain(s) (*see also* Painful), hand, *see* Pain, limb, upper, hand
R20.2      Paresthesia, *see also* Disturbance(s), sensation (cold) (heat) (localization) (tactile discrimination) (texture) (vibratory), skin, paresthesia
Z33.1      Pregnancy (childbirth) (labor) (puerperium), incidental finding

**1.241.** A04.7      Colitis (acute) (catarrhal) (chronic (noninfective) (hemorrhagic), Clostridium difficile
E86.0      Dehydration
I73.9      Disease, diseased, peripheral vascular NOS

**1.242.** F32.9      Depression (acute) (mental), major
Z63.4      Bereavement (uncomplicated)

**1.243.** E66.01    Obesity, due to, excessive calories, morbid
I10         Hypertension, hypertensive (accelerated) (benign) (essential) (idiopathic) (malignant) (systemic)
E78.0      Hypercholesterolemia (essential) (familial) (hereditary) (primary) (pure)

**1.244.** H66.003  Otitis (acute), media (hemorrhagic) (staphylococcal) (streptococcal), suppurative, acute
J06.9      Infection, infected, infective (opportunistic) respiratory (tract), upper (acute)

**1.245.** E11.43    Diabetes, diabetic (mellitus) (sugar) type 2, with, gastroparesis
K31.84    Gastroparesis
Z79.4      Therapy, drug, long-term (current) (prophylactic), insulin <u>or</u>
Long-term (current) (prophylactic) drug therapy (use of), insulin

**1.246.** N18.6      Disease, diseased, renal (chronic) (functional) (pelvis), end-stage (failure)
Z99.2      Dependence (on) (syndrome), on, renal dialysis (hemodialysis) (peritoneal) <u>or</u> Presence (of), arterial-venous shunt (dialysis)

**1.247.** C67.3      Neoplasm Table, by site, bladder (urinary), malignant, primary site, wall, anterior
N40.0      Hypertrophy, hypertrophic, prostate – *see* Enlargement, enlarged, prostate
Z92.21    History, personal (of), chemotherapy for neoplastic condition

**1.248.** M15.0      Arthritis, arthritic (acute) (chronic) (nonpyogenic) (subacute) degenerative – *see* Osteoarthritis
Osteoarthritis, generalized, primary

M47.817    Osteoarthritis, spine – *see* Spondylosis
Spondylosis, without myelopathy or radiculopathy, lumbosacral region

I25.10      Arteriosclerosis, arteriosclerotic (diffuse) (obliterans) (of) (senile) (with calcification), coronary (artery)

I10         Hypertension, hypertensive (accelerated) (benign) (essential) (idiopathic) (malignant) (systemic)

**1.249. Answer, First visit:**

E30.0      Delay, delayed, puberty (constitutional)

Z60.4      Problem (with) (related to), social, exclusion and rejection

**Answer, Second visit:**

E23.0      Deficiency, deficient, growth hormone (idiopathic) (isolated)

**1.250.** T83.51XA   Complication(s) (from) (of), catheter (device), urethral, indwelling, infection and inflammation

N39.0      Infection, infected, infective (opportunistic), urinary (tract)

B96.20    Infection, infected, infective (opportunistic), Escherichia (E) coli, as cause of disease classified elsewhere

**1.251.** I13.2      Failure, failed, heart (acute) (senile) (sudden), hypertensive – *see* Hypertension, heart. Hypertension, hypertensive (accelerated) (benign) (essential) (idiopathic) (malignant) (systemic), heart (disease) (conditions in I51.4-I51.9 due to hypertension), with kidney disease (chronic) – *see* Hypertension, cardiorenal (chronic). Hypertension, cardiorenal, with heart failure, with stage 5 or end stage renal disease

I50.9      Failure, heart (acute) (senile) (sudden), congestive (compensated) (decompensated)

N18.5      Disease, diseased, kidney (functional) (pelvis, chronic, stage 5)

## *Hospital Outpatient Cases*

**1.252.** A60.01    Herpes, herpesvirus, herpetic, penis

A60.02    Herpes, herpesvirus, herpetic, scrotum

R94.5      Findings, abnormal, inconclusive, without diagnosis, function study, liver

Z21         HIV, positive, seropositive

F11.229    Dependence (on) (syndrome), heroin – *see* Dependence, drug, opioid, with, intoxication

Z72.51    Problem (with) (related to), life style, high risk sexual behavior (heterosexual)

**1.253.** Z51.11    Chemotherapy (session) (for), cancer

C25.7      Neoplasm Table, by site, pancreas, neck, malignant, primary site

E86.0      Dehydration

R11.2      Nausea, with vomiting

T45.1X5A   Table of Drugs and Chemicals, Anticancer agents NEC, adverse effect

**1.254.** D57.219   Disease, diseased, sickle cell, Hb-C with crisis (vasoocclusive pain)

E11.9      Diabetes, diabetic (mellitus) (sugar), type 2

Z63.8      Inadequate, inadequacy, family support

**1.255.** D50.0      Anemia (essential) (general) (hemoglobin deficiency) (infantile) (primary) (profound), blood loss (chronic)

|  | E11.9 | Diabetes, diabetic (mellitus) (sugar), type 2 |
|---|---|---|
|  | I25.10 | Disease, diseased, coronary (artery) *see* – disease, heart, ischemic, atherosclerotic; Disease, heart, ischemic, atherosclerotic (of) |
|  | Z95.1 | Status (post), aortocoronary bypass |
|  | Z57.5 | Exposure (to) (*see also* contact, with), occupational toxic agents (gases) (liquids) (solids) (vapors) in industry NEC |
| **1.256.** | P28.81 | Arrest, arrested, respiratory, newborn |
|  | P29.81 | Arrest, arrested, cardiac, newborn |
|  | P07.18 | Low, birth weight, with weight of, 2000–2499 grams |
| **1.257.** | R07.9 | Pain(s) (*see also* Painful), chest (central) |
|  | R06.02 | Short, shortening, shortness, breath |
|  | I10 | Hypertension, hypertensive (accelerated) (benign) (essential) (idiopathic) (malignant) (systemic) |
|  | E10.65 | Diabetes, diabetic (mellitus) (sugar), out of control – code to Diabetes, by type, with hyperglycemia. Diabetes, diabetic, type 1, with hyperglycemia |
|  | E10.51 | Diabetes, diabetic (mellitus) (sugar), type 1, with peripheral angiopathy |
| **1.258.** | T25.211A | Burn (electricity) (flame) (hot gas, liquid or hot object) (radiation) (steam) (thermal), ankle, right, second degree |
|  | X12.XXXA | Index to External Causes, Burn, burned, burning (accidental) (by) (from) (on), hot liquid |
|  | Y92.010 | Index to External Causes, Place of occurrence, residence (non-institutional) (private), house, single family, kitchen |
|  | Y93.G3 | Index to External Causes, Activity (involving) (of victim at time of event), cooking and baking |
|  | Y99.8 | Index to External Causes, External cause status, leisure activity |
| **1.259.** | K57.92 | Diverticulitis (acute) |
|  | Z80.0 | History, family (of), malignant neoplasm (of), gastrointestinal tract <u>or</u> History, family (of), malignant neoplasm (of), digestive organ |
|  | I10 | Hypertension, hypertensive (accelerated) (benign) (essential) (idiopathic) (malignant) (systemic) |
| **1.260.** | H05.012 | Cellulitis (diffuse) (phlegmonous) (septic) (suppurative), orbit, orbital |
|  | H00.024 | Hordeolum (eyelid) (externum) (recurrent), internum, left, upper |
| **1.261.** | R09.1 | Pleurisy (acute) (adhesive) (chronic) (costal) (diaphragmatic) (double) (dry) (fibrinous) (fibrous) (interlobar) (latent) (plastic) (primary) (residual) (sicca) (sterile) (subacute) (unresolved) |
|  | B97.89 | Infection, infected, infective (opportunistic) virus, viral, as a cause of disease classified elsewhere |
|  | G35 | Sclerosis, sclerotic, multiple (brain stem) (cerebral) (generalized) (spinal cord) |
| **1.262.** | M12.39 | Rheumatism (articular) (neuralgic) (nonarticular), palindromic, multiple site |
|  | N39.46 | Incontinence, urge, and stress (female) (male) |
| **1.263.** | G44.001 | Headache, cluster, intractable |

**1.264.** Z52.3      Donor (organ or tissue), bone, marrow
R50.82      Fever (inanition) (of unknown origin) (persistent) (with chills) (with rigor), postoperative
R11.2      Nausea, with vomiting

**1.265.** K80.51      Jaundice (yellow), obstructive – *see also* Obstruction, bile duct
Obstruction, obstructed, obstructive, bile duct or passage (common) (hepatic) (noncalculous), with calculus
R00.0      Tachycardia

**1.266.** N76.4      Abscess (connective tissue) (embolic) (fistulous) (infective) (metastatic) (multiple) (pernicious) (pyogenic) (septic), labium (majus) (minus) <u>or</u> Abscess, vulva
Z88.2      History, personal (of), allergy (to) sulfonamides

**1.267.** J20.9      Bronchitis (diffuse) (fibrinous) (hypostatic) (infective) (membranous) (with tracheitis), acute or subacute (with bronchospasm or obstruction)
D86.0      Sarcoidosis, lung
M25.50      Arthralgia, *see also* Pain, joint
R03.0      Elevated, elevation, blood pressure reading (incidental) (isolated) (nonspecific), no diagnosis of hypertension

**1.268.** J06.9      Infection, infected, infective (opportunistic) respiratory (tract), upper (acute), viral NOS
D70.9      Neutropenia, neutropenic (chronic) (genetic) (idiopathic) (immune) (infantile) (malignant) (pernicious) (splenic)
M31.30      Granulomatosis, Wegener's

**1.269.** H04.553      Stenosis, stenotic, nasolacrimal duct, *see also* Stenosis, lacrimal duct
Q93.5      Syndrome, Angelman

**1.270.** I49.3      Contractions(s), contracture, contracted, premature, ventricular

**1.271.** K56.1      Intussusception (bowel) (colon) (enteric) (ileocecal) (ileocolic) (intestine) (rectum)
K52.9      Gastroenteritis (acute) (chronic) (noninfectious)
R68.11      Excess, excessive, excessively crying of infant

**1.272.** K02.9      Caries, dental
F88      Delay, delayed, development, global
Z94.4      Transplant(ed) (status), liver

# AHIMA ICD-10 Products

**Available at www.ahimastore.org**

## Books from AHIMA Press
- *Implementing ICD-10-CM/PCS for Hospitals* (AC201009)
- *Pocket Guide of ICD-10-CM and ICD-10-PCS* (AC203010)
- *ICD-10-CM and ICD-10-PCS Preview*, Second Edition (AC206009)
- *ICD-10-CM and ICD-10-PCS Preview Exercises*, Second Edition (AC216011)
- *ICD-10-CM Coder Training Manual 2013* (AC206813)
- *ICD-10-PCS Coder Training Manual 2013* (AC207813)
- *Transitioning to ICD-10-CM/PCS: The Essential Guide to General Equivalence Mappings (GEMs)* (AC202810)
- *Root Operations: Key to Procedure Coding in ICD-10-PCS* (AC211010)
- *ICD-10-PCS: An Applied Approach* (AC201111)
- *Basic ICD-10-CM/PCS Coding Exercises,* Fourth Edition (AC210512)
- *ICD-10-CM and ICD-9-CM Diagnostic Coding and Reimbursement for Physician*
- *Services,* 2013 (AC201212)
- *Basic ICD-10-CM/PCS and ICD-9-CM Coding,* 2012 (AC200511)
- *Clinical Coding Workout with Answers,* 2013 Update (AC201514)

## AHIMA Online Education
AHIMA offers a complete program of online ICD-10 training for organizational and non-coding staff, acute-care coders, and specialty coding settings
- ICD-10-CM Overview
- ICD-10-PCS Overview
- Comprehensive online ICD-10-CM (26 hours)
- Comprehensive online ICD-10-PCS (24 hours)
- Coding Proficiency Assessments
- ICD-10-CM Coding Assessment
- ICD-10-PCS Coding Assessment
- ICD-10 A&P System Coding Assessments

## AHIMA Meetings, Audio Seminars, and Webinars
- Annual ICD-10/Computer-Assisted Summit
- Academy for ICD-10-CM/PCS Trainers (multiple dates and locations throughout the year)
- Coder Workforce Training for ICD-10 (multiple dates and locations throughout the year)
- Private Academies (Contact AHIMA's Business Innovation Group.)
- Annual Clinical Coding Meeting
- AHIMA Annual Convention and Exhibits

AHIMA is constantly developing products and resources to meet the needs of HIM professionals. Check ahima.org for updates and announcements of new products.

## Code Books from Optum
- *ICD-10-CM: The Complete Official Draft Code Set* 2013 (VC209113)
- *ICD-10-PCS: The Complete Official Draft Code Set* 2013 (VC209213)